CANADIAN MEDICAL LIVES NO. 4

CLARENCE HINCKS

MENTAL HEALTH CRUSADER

CHARLES G. ROLAND

Series Editor: T.P. Morley, M.D.

Hannah Institute
&
Dundurn Press
Toronto and Oxford
1990

Design and Production: JAQ
Copy Editor: Patti Giovannini
Printing and Binding: Gagné Printing Ltd., Louiseville, Quebec, Canada

Care has been taken to trace the ownership of copyright material used in the text, including the illustrations. The author and publisher welcome any information enabling them to rectify any reference or credit in subsequent editions.

J. Kirk Howard, Publisher

Canadian Cataloguing in Publication Data

Roland, Charles G., 1933-
Clarence Hincks : mental health crusader

(Canadian medical lives series)
ISBN 1-55002-048-X

1. Hincks, Clarence, 1885-1964. 2. Mental health - Canada - History. 3. Canadian Mental Health Association - Biography. 4. Physicians - Canada - Biography. I. Title. II. Series: Canadian medical lives.

RA790.7.H5R6 1990 616.8'092 C90-095156-7

Dundurn Press Limited
2181 Queen Street East
Suite 301
Toronto, Canada
M4E 1E5

Dundurn Distribution Limited
73 Lime Walk
Headington
Oxford, England
OX3 7AD

CANADIAN MEDICAL LIVES SERIES

The story of the Hannah Institute for the History of Medicine has been told by John B. Neilson and G.R. Paterson in *Associated Medical Services, Incorporated: A History* (1987). With the creation of the Institute the AMS endowed it with funds, capability and responsibility to develop and disseminate a body of medical history hitherto hidden in the country's memory.

A grants and personnel support program enables the Institute through medical, social and political historians to become a powerful influence in the rapidly expanding interest accorded to medical history. A chair in the history of medicine is supported at each of the five Ontario medical schools.

Originally the Institute's support was limited to Ontario, but it has now been extended to medical historical work in any part of Canada.

Dr. Donald R. Wilson, President of Associated Medical Services, persuaded the Board that the Hannah Institute should launch a series of biographies of those who, as yet unsung, had made major contributions in the broad field of Canadian medicine during their lifetime. The Institute also had in mind for the series members of the nursing profession, particularly those who had pioneered public health services, as well as workers in related fields.

Professor Roland's story of Hincks introduces Canadians to the man who, more than any other, rescued mental illness and emotional disturbance from the darkness of the past and brought it into the light of public scrutiny.

The next volumes in the Canadian Medical Lives Series include Emily Stowe (Mary Fryer), Mahlon W. Locke (Robert Jackson), Francis A. C. Scrimger (Suzanne Kingsmill), R. G. Ferguson (Stuart Houston), J. C. B. Grant (C.L.N. Robinson), and Earle B. Scarlett (Bill Mussellwhite).

There is no shortage of meritorious subjects. Willing and capable authors are difficult to acquire. The Institute is therefore deeply grateful to the early authors who have already committed their time and skill to the series.

T.P. Morley
Series Editor
1990

CANADIAN MEDICAL LIVES SERIES

1. *Duncan Graham* by Robert B. Kerr and Douglas Waugh*
2. *Bill Mustard* by Marilyn Dunlop*
3. *Joe Doupe* by Terence Moore*
4. *Clarence Hincks* by Charles G. Roland*
5. *Francis A.C. Scrimger, V.C.,* by Suzanne Kingsmill
6. *Emily Stowe* by Mary Beacock Fryer
7. *William Canniff* by Heather MacDougall
8. *James M. Langstaff* by Jacalyn M. Duffin
9. *Earle B. Scarlett* by Bill Musselwhite
10. *Marguerite Carr-Harris, RN,* by Meryn Stuart
11. *Mahlon W. Locke* by Robert Jackson
12. *Wallace Graham* by Joan Hollobon
13. *Maude Abbott* by Douglas Waugh
14. *J.C.B. Grant* by C.L.N. Robinson
15. *William Boyd* by Ian Carr
16. *William Carson* by H.H. Nixon
17. *R.G. Ferguson* by Stuart Houston
18. *William T. Aikins* by Charles M. Godfrey
19. *R.M. Bucke* by Helene Fallen

*published

CANADIAN MEDICAL LIVES NO. 4

CLARENCE HINCKS

MENTAL HEALTH CRUSADER

CHARLES G. ROLAND

Series Editor: T.P. Morley, M.D.

For my daughter

Kathleen Siobhan Roland Ruben

who, quite unconsciously, has done much over the years
to improve the author's mental equilibrium

TABLE OF CONTENTS

	PREFACE	8
	PROLOGUE	9
1.	THE EARLY YEARS	11
2.	INTERNSHIP AND FIRST PRACTICE	21
3.	ESTABLISHING IN TORONTO	26
4.	THE CANADIAN NATIONAL COMMITTEE FOR MENTAL HYGIENE	39
5.	ASPIRATIONS AND ACCOMPLISHMENTS	45
6.	BLOWING UP THE PARLIAMENT BUILDINGS AND OTHER PROGRESS	60
7.	NEW DIRECTIONS FOR THE CNCMH	77
8.	TRIP TO EUROPE, 1925-26	83
9.	DOUBLE DUTY, CANADA AND THE USA	96
10.	THE SECOND WORLD WAR	104
11.	THE POST-WAR YEARS	109
12.	CLARE HINCKS AND HIS FAMILY	115
13.	THE SUMMING-UP	120
	ENDNOTES	124
	BIBLIOGRAPHY	125
	LIST OF ILLUSTRATIONS	126
	INDEX	127

PREFACE

THIS SHORT BIOGRAPHY is intended as a tribute to a most remarkable man, Clarence Meredith Hincks (1885-1964). Doctor Hincks took a major role in founding the Canadian National Committee for Mental Hygiene in 1918; this organization later became the Canadian Mental Health Association. This is not a history of the Association, however, although much information about its activities is included here.

Some anecdotal autobiographical notes, dictated by Clare Hincks in 1960 and 1961, formed the starting point for this book. Where possible I have checked the details of these recollections although, given their nature, this is a difficult and uncertain task. Throughout the text portions of these notes — direct quotes from Dr. Hincks — appear in an indented format.

I gratefully acknowledge the assistance of many people in preparing this biography; none of these persons shares in any way my responsibility for the accuracy of the text and the statements and opinions contained herein. Professor Cyril Greenland and Dr. Jack Griffin, Clare's protégé and successor as General Director of the CMHA, deserve particular thanks for their long-term encouragement and co-operation, particularly during the preparation of a much earlier version of this manuscript; and Audrey M. Wilson and David Michaels for providing photographs of the C.M. Hincks Institute and the C.M. Hincks Treatment Centre. Others who granted interviews or wrote lengthy letters of reminiscence about Clare (mostly in the 1960s) include the following: the late Mrs. Marjorie Keyes Hincks, Miss Margaret Hincks, Mrs. Barbara Hincks Toivanen, Reverend N. William Hincks, Dr. Gordon Bates, Professor W.G. Blatz, Colonel H. Edmund Bullis, George E. Bushnell, Dr. D. Ewen Cameron, Dr. Brock Chisholm, Dr. Gerald Cosgrove, A.L. Crease, Miss Margaret Davis, Dr. Edward Fidlar, G.H. Gooderham, Prof. Cyril Greenland, Dr. G. Edward Hall, Dr. Archibald Huntsman, D.M. LeBourdais, Dr. J.M. MacEachran, Mrs. E. Lloyd (Cringan) Marrow, Morgan Parmenter, Dr. T.A. Pincock, Dr. H.B. Spaulding, Dr. George Stevenson, and Dr. G.S. Stevenson.

C.G.R.
Hamilton, Ontario

PROLOGUE

On a day in 1910, in a small office in a west Toronto school, a young man and a child faced each other across a desk. There was nothing particularly dramatic in their confrontation. The young man, a school physician, regularly examined children at this and other Toronto schools. Nor was the child unique. Indeed, this was a part of the problem: the youngster resembled many others in the school system — children who did poorly in school, lagging behind their age group until they ended up discouraged, awkward, and oversized compared with others in their class. Teachers often criticized them for inattentiveness, or laziness, or badness, or stupidity.

Sometimes, when examining these students, he found a disease or condition to explain their difficulty. More often he found nothing. Occasionally he saw a child who was plainly feeble-minded, but this was rare; such children were seldom sent to school. The children this physician puzzled over looked like other children, yet were different. Were they lazy? Or bad? Or stupid? How could he be sure?

The man was Clarence Meredith Hincks, a 25-year-old physician — and perplexed. This is his story, the life of the man who, for over 50 years was dedicated to helping people like the child on the other side of the desk.

What sort of man was he? Can we analyze some of the factors that united to produce Clare Hincks, founder of the Canadian Mental Health Association?

Clare was an only child, frail and much fussed over. All his adult life he suffered from a recurrent mental disorder that produced frequent episodes of incapacitation. He became totally involved in his work in mental hygiene; his wife and his children were largely ignored for long periods while he travelled throughout North America. He did not receive the best of postgraduate training in psychiatry, and was probably not an outstanding clinician. Indeed, when he became Medical Director of the Canadian National Committee for Mental Hygiene in 1924, his appointment was conditional on his acquiring further postgraduate training.

Despite these deficiencies, if they were deficiencies, Clare Hincks acquired a reputation for hard work, inspiration, and a fantastic ability to raise money for mental hygiene. From 1919 until his death from liver cancer in 1964, Clare Hincks served the only love of his professional life, the mental health movement. On the day he entered hospital for the last time he worked on a speech entitled "How You and I can Promote Mental Health" — an apt conclusion to the career of one of Canada's most successful promoters.

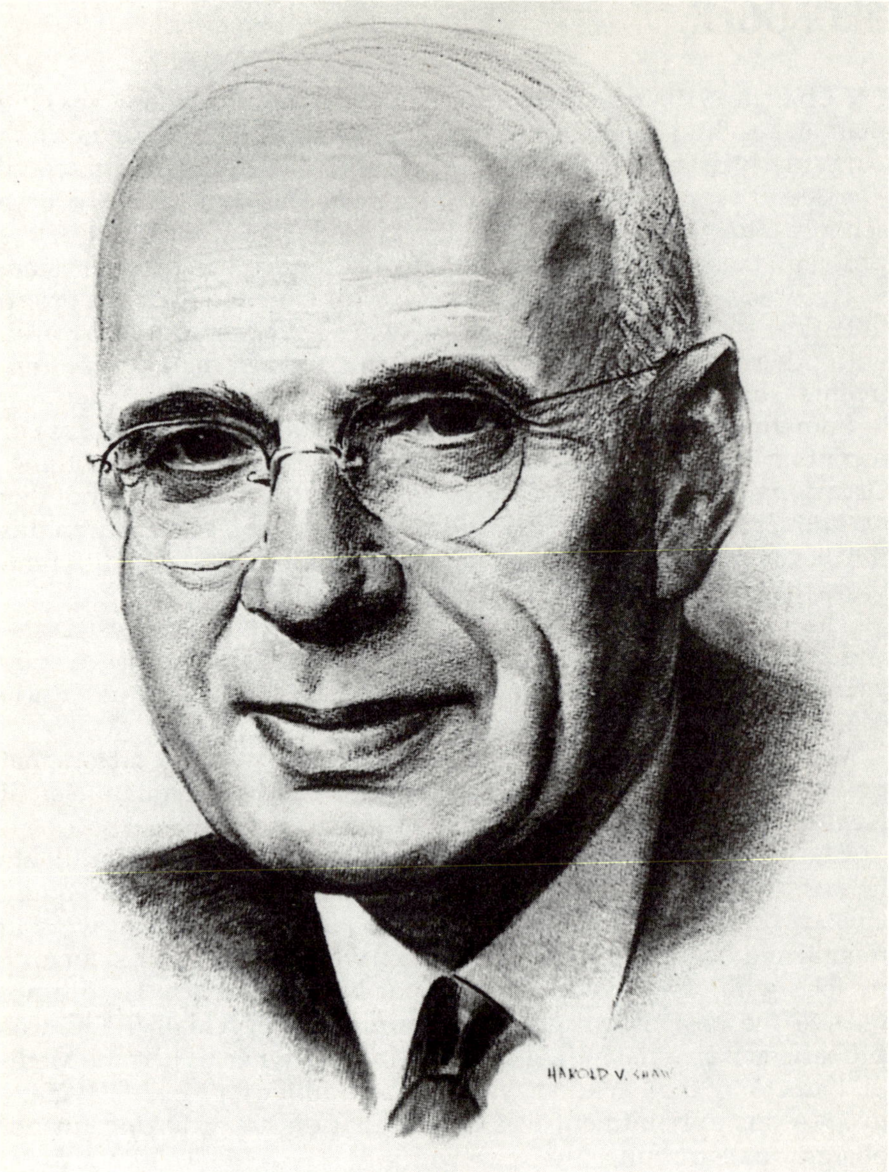
HAROLD V. SHAW

Chapter One

THE EARLY YEARS

THE FARMLANDS AND SMALL TOWNS of Ontario have contributed generously to the ranks of eminent Canadian physicians. Among the many distinguished doctors born or raised in these bucolic surroundings are William Osler, Frederick Banting, Duncan Graham, Richard Maurice Bucke, and Clarence Meredith Hincks. Like Osler and Bucke, Hincks was the son of a clergyman.

St. Marys, Ontario, was typical of hundreds of small towns dotting the countryside in 1885; it served as the focus for a few square miles of cultivated lands. Near London and the now famous Stratford, farmers of the area enjoyed relative prosperity. Hard work could produce an adequate living and at least some luxury. One luxury which distinguished St. Marys from a lot of other small Ontario towns 100 years ago was a Methodist minister by the name of William Henry Hincks, father of Clarence Hincks.

Clarence (Clare) Hincks was born in St. Marys on 6 April 1885, an only child of quite exceptional parents. Mrs. Hincks, who became a dominant figure in the life of her son, was a former school teacher who had assisted talented pupils in obtaining higher education. One such pupil, fourteen years her junior, had been William Henry Hincks. As Clare relates:

> [My father] was a poor immigrant boy, and my mother financed him through the university on the condition that he would never ask her to marry him, because as she said: "I am old enough to be your mother." She made the great mistake, however, of sending him a postcard of congratulations upon his graduation in theology and law. On receipt of this card, my father, who by this time had become engaged to another girl, broke off the engagement and exclaimed to a classmate: "Mattie Greene is worth a dozen of my present girl and I am taking the next train to Hamilton to marry her."

He promptly did so.

Clare Hincks's father was a Cockney, born in 1859. After emigrating to Canada with his parents in the 1870s he finished high school in Hamilton, Ontario, and attended Victoria University in Cobourg, where he received encouragement and financial help from his future wife. After graduation and ordination in 1884, Reverend Hincks began what was to become a distinguished career as a Methodist clergyman. A brilliant speaker and an inspired pastor, he was beloved by his parishioners for his sound counsel and generous assistance in resolving their difficulties. From his first charge at Nissouri, near St. Marys, he went to Preston in 1887, Stratford in 1890, Owen Sound in 1893, and to Toronto in 1896. The remainder of his professional life was centred in Toronto, where he had a total of eight charges before retirement in 1929.

Clare was a thin, frail child, believed to have been a victim of rickets. His family physician had reported that he might not live past the age of fifteen, yet during his elementary and high school years Clare spent summer holidays at Windermere on Lake Rosseau, and while at university he spent four months there each year, two working and two on holiday. In those days the benefits of fresh air and sunlight were just beginning to be understood. They worked well for Clare Hincks, who once said, "In my opinion I owe my long life to Muskoka."

Many of Clare's reminiscences of childhood relate to his vacations at Muskoka. It was there that he also had the opportunity to design one of his first successful promotions. J.W. Bengough, the political cartoonist, was touring the area and charging admission to nightly demonstrations of his art. Since business was unsatisfactory, he accepted Clare's offer to boost attendance at Windermere. Hincks the huckster, amplified by a megaphone, produced the desired result and Bengough hired him for the remainder of his tour in the Muskoka area.

Because of his frail physique Clare was never active in the strenuous team sports most boys enjoy. At one school event, however, a "slow bicycle race" was announced, with first prize going to the student who took the longest time to cycle a prescribed course. Clare entered and won, enjoying what may be his only moment of glory in competitive sport. Later, however, when in medical practice, he became an enthusiastic sailor and canoeist. Clare embarked on three- and four-day canoe trips to Georgian Bay every summer for many years, travelling with his close friend, George Anderson, or his future brother-in-law, Norman Millman, and sleeping under his canoe at night.

On one such excursion in the 1920s, Clare and three friends set out from Windermere on what was to be a lengthy canoe trip. They had just lost sight of the Hincks' cottage when a raging storm struck and they were forced to paddle ashore to the Muskoka Country Club near Port Carling. The surroundings there were so congenial that they stayed four days, playing cards, eating, drinking, and sleeping in comfort before finally paddling home to regale wives and families with tales of peril and adventure — until the bills arrived.

Clare never lost his love of the water. His only son, William, recalls his own delight when, as a boy, he was judged sufficiently adept to crew on his father's racing sloop *Sewanee*.

Clare's ease in making friends may have grown from the frequent moves demanded of a minister and his family. He had vivid memories of attending tearful farewell services one week and becoming firmly established in a new parish the next, with dozens of new friends. His gregarious nature was to be well suited to the promotion of mental hygiene throughout North America.

Clare admitted openly that he was thoroughly spoiled by his mother. Although it may be more accurate to say that he was indulged by her, he was also stimulated by this remarkable woman. She served Clare and his father faithfully, showering them with affection and making it clear that she considered them quite exceptional.

> My mother's delusion that we were both great was shared by us and accounts for each of us in our chosen professions facing the world with supreme confidence and taking chances without the slightest fear of defeat .... With mother on our side, we felt invincible.

Of course, life for Clare was not all canoe trips, summer holidays and maternal indulgence. Through the public and high school years Clare managed his studies with ease, having the advantage of professional coaching from his mother. He was ready for university at age 15, but, by regulation, could not be admitted until he was 16, so in the year 1900, the family took advantage of Clare's year out of school and travelled to Europe. The luxury of travel was not easy for a minister's family to afford. For many years the Hinckses had hoarded their "marriage" and "wedding" money. In the family parlance, a "marriage" was, by definition, a ceremony for which the Reverend Mr. Hincks received less than five dollars; anything more constituted a "wedding." By nursing their small fund carefully the family was able to spend almost four months overseas. Unfortunately no details of the trip now exist so we are left to surmise its effect on Clare. Certainly it was the last major indulgence his family allowed him, for when they returned, Clare enrolled at the University of Toronto.

While still in his mid-teens, a difficult stage in any youngster's life, Clare was cut loose from his mother's apron strings. After 16 years of physical and emotional dependency, he was suddenly forced to make his own decisions about university and his future. This experience almost certainly contributed to Clare's first episode of emotional illness, an affliction that would recur throughout his life and which would play a prominent role in directing his future career in psychiatry.

At the University of Toronto he enrolled in biology and physics, primarily, it seems, because this course required a minimum of mathematics — not an area that was particularly strong with Clare. After three months of study, Clare's class was presented with a special option by the university; they could obtain degrees in both Arts and Medicine after only six years of study. Customarily, seven or eight years of study was required to receive both degrees. This offer appealed to the class of seven: Archie Huntsman, Cooper Cole, Fletcher McPhedran, Ernest Henderson, Eddie Fidlar, Ross Mulholland, and Clare Hincks, and they all accepted. The group graduated in 1907, at the same time as the larger, regular class of that year. Members of the other class included Gordon Bates, who would become prominent in the field of social medicine, and Alan Roy Dafoe, later famous as the practitioner who delivered Mrs. Dionne of the quintuplets.

Clare categorized himself as a mediocre student, placing part of the blame on his inability to study after eight o'clock in the evening because he became unalterably drowsy at that time. Since lectures and laboratory work filled the days until about six o'clock, little time remained for study.

Clare was impressed, however, by many of his teachers at the University of Toronto, particularly Dr. W.P. Caven (1861-1943), Mr. I.H. Cameron (1854-1934), and Professor Ramsay Wright (1852-1933).

William Proudfoot Caven was an outstanding physician in Toronto. Like Clare, he was born in St. Marys and his father was a minister. Caven drilled his students into writing painstaking and complete medical histories to cover all facets of the patient's life, habits, family, and occupation. This exercise would aid Clare when he began his work in psychiatry, since in no field of medicine is a clear and complete case history more important. In Clare's opinion Caven was one of the most talented physicians ever to practise in Toronto.

Mr. I.H. Cameron was the Professor of Surgery. Following a tradition of British surgeons which is upheld to this day, he prided himself in the designation "Mister," not "Doctor."

> He had a goatee, and when he laughed ... his goatee would bob up and down. One day when his lecture was over, I walked down the steps at the front of the medical building and imitated Mr. Cameron's laugh.
>
> At this point, a hand was placed on my shoulder; the hand belonged to the man I was imitating. Mr. Cameron asked me my name. I said: "Hincks." He replied: "I'm sorry to hear that because at one time in the history of this University we needed an additional lecturer in biology. We had two applicants for this post. One man's name was Hincks and we lost the great Thomas Huxley." My reply was rather a rude one. "If Huxley had come to Toronto, he might not have developed his great talents or made his great contribution." At this Mr. Cameron pondered and then admitted that I might be right.

At any rate, Cameron seemed to bear Hincks no ill will for his impertinence, since Clare took top marks in his oral examination in surgery.

Ramsay Wright, Professor of Biology, was the first to hold the post in Toronto. He was a tall, fine looking man and a lucid, charming lecturer who, in spite of being Canadian, spoke with an extreme Oxford accent that he had acquired while studying in England. Although in most men this would have been considered a distasteful affectation, apparently this was not true of Professor Wright. His teaching inspired in Clare a love of biology that he retained through the years.

Clare also remembered many distinguished visitors to the campus while he was a student, one of the most memorable being the great Canadian expatriate physician, Sir William Osler. At that time Professor of Medicine at Johns Hopkins University, Osler was considered the greatest physician in the world at the turn of the century. He and his colleagues had ushered in the new scientific method, coordinating teaching at the patient's bedside with the burgeoning advances of biochemistry, bacteriology, pathology, and pharmacology. Osler's textbook, *The Principles and Practice of Medicine*, was, in its successive editions, the standard work in most corners of the world.

Clare was privileged as a student to hear Osler speak on several occasions. In an introductory lecture to Clare's class in October, 1903, Sir William gave his famed address, "The Master Word in Medicine," in which he advocated the word *work* as a motto for medical students. In this and other lectures, Clare was notably impressed and inspired by this great man.[1]

> I found Sir William Osler to be captivating, human, profound, a great philosopher, a man one would never forget. I still remember a remark he made in one of his lectures: "The task of medicine is to bring in the medicine of the future." In other words, medicine must never become smug and stand still.

Clare's interest in academics by no means excluded him from the games that students are apt to play.

Directly across from the medical school was the School of Practical Science where the engineers studied. The two institutions were bitter rivals and Clare described several battles that took place between them. On one occasion a medical student was caught by the engineers, stripped to the waist and painted with the engineering colours. In retaliation, an unwary engineering student was caught and treated to a "shampoo" with ground human liver and Canada balsam, a cement from the sap of the balsam fir used to seal specimens on microscope slides. The only way to remove such a horrible mixture was by shaving all the hair in the affected area.

Similar tales abound in every college graduate's repertoire; one of Clare's classmates, Archie Huntsman, has related a companion story, dating it about 1901:

> ... the Meds were just across Taddle Creek Road from the (engineering) School men in their red brick building. The scraps between Meds and School were not infrequent

> and were more exciting than our Freshmen hustles. They were usually started by the School men, perhaps as a relief from the monotony of their work with the "two-foot rule."
>
> One that occurred in our first year, in October of 1901, seemed to be the best. The Meds were definitely victorious, but the School maintained that this was due to most unequal numbers (350 vs 200). Some School men had in the dark hours painted the School colours on the flagpole that stood near the sidewalk in front of the Anatomical wing of the Biology [Building]. A day or so later, they removed the pole by sawing it off. Thus the scrap *had* to be.
>
> The Meds assembled for the fray in full force at 2:30 pm, and marched from the Biology to the campus. Dean Reeve pleaded with them to desist, but without effect. The flagpole was between the two forces, and, under superior medical power, [it was] moved across the road and down into the ravine between Library and Biology. A window in the latter was opened for the pole to enter, which had to be sawn in two to get all of it in and close the window.
>
> With victory, the Meds meted out the usual punishment to such foes as could be captured. The use of water in "tapping" prisoners was common to both antagonists, but in place of the inks used by the School men, the Meds used from their laboratories various tissue stains for permanent colouring and Canada balsam for its adhesiveness and relative insolubility. These were applied to such parts of the anatomy of the captives as could be bared, the more objectionable the better. Some of the School men were even hauled upstairs to the dissecting room at the very top and subjected to nameless indignities. The School men suffered more than this, because they found after the scrap that the authorities had given them a holiday by locking their building with many of their hats and coats inside. Students could be seen dodging their way home, hatless, coatless, and in a few cases, we understand, shirtless.

Clare was a victim himself on one occasion when acting as a supernumerary in a performance of *Aïda* at the Princess Theatre. His part involved playing a trumpet, and at one point in the performance he put his instrument to his lips when no music was being played. At the same moment, an engineer in the audience surreptitiously blew his own trumpet. Clare was blamed for the mishap and thrown out of the show without his fifty cents, the usual payment for his part in the performance.

The Princess Theatre was one of Clare's favourite haunts as a student. For twenty-five cents he could sit in the top balcony and see celebrities like Sarah Bernhardt, E.S. Willard, Sir Henry Irving, Julia Marlowe, Forbes Robertson, Robert B. Montell, and John Barrymore. At Massey Hall he enjoyed Paderewski, Nordica, Calvi, Fritz Kreisler, Heifitz, Pavlova, Luisa Tetrazzini, and the Philadelphia Orchestra.

Clare also enjoyed weekly visits to Shea's Theatre for an evening of vaudeville and other attractions. On one visit, Clare heard a monologue by James T. Corbett, who had defeated John L. Sullivan for the heavyweight championship of the world. After the performance Clare met "Gentleman Jim" at the stage door and invited him to give a boxing demonstration at the University gymnasium. Corbett accepted and later gave a memorable "clinic" to the university boxing team. During his presentation he emphasized, among other things, the importance of footwork and body motion. To illustrate, he stood in the ring and invited members of the University team to enter the ring and attempt to hit him. Corbett held his arms at his sides and did nothing but sway his body and step gracefully from side to side. Not one of the team members landed a blow.

We know little of Clare's social activities within the university except that he became a member of Psi Delta Psi fraternity, although there is no mention of this in his autobiographical notes. None of Clare's surviving classmates has retained any distinctive memories of him as a student except that he was younger than many of his companions and apparently shy.

So Clare's college days followed the pattern familiar to generations of students—work and play, the latter the more memorable. However, one definite and decisive difference existed for Clare. During his introductory year at university, he experienced the first of his "attacks."

This attack, occurring at the age of 16, was the first episode of what would become an almost annual problem until 1959, the year of his retirement. Clare believed the cessation of his attacks in that year was due to the removal of the tensions of his work. Whatever the reason, there is little question that these bouts of mental illness were of major importance in shaping his attitude to and interest in mental health:

> I can remember the circumstances of this first attack very vividly. At the time, I was playing bridge at the home of one of my pals on St. George Street, Toronto. I had been feeling

> in fine health and excellent spirits, and then, during the game, a sudden change came over me. Without physical pain, my world cracked up. I lost all interest in the game I was playing. I felt completely different from my former self. My interest in friends and life itself completely vanished. Although I could talk, I did not want to communicate with anyone. I was not severely depressed, but was completely inert. Those around me were laughing but I could not enter into their gay spirits. Indeed, I marvelled that anyone in the world could laugh. I had become in a fraction of a second a vegetable.

Clare didn't know what was wrong. He went home to bed, and since he was unable to concentrate on anything he decided to stay there until he felt better. The family decided not to call a doctor but to let nature take its course. Within two weeks, as Clare gradually felt normal again, he resumed his college work.

It requires little imagination to perceive the impact of this strange event on a 16-year-old boy. It is demoralizing to undergo a complete change of personality, and often more frightening than a physical illness with a specific cause. Clare himself labelled his illness a neurosis, yet, far from considering the manifestations of neuroses and psychoses as detrimental, he thought of them as devices of nature to give the mind a rest and thus to give the individual an opportunity to regain inner strength.

Whatever their real significance, these periods of illness had no adverse effect on Clare's academic progress. After receiving a BA degree in 1905, he graduated MD in 1907.

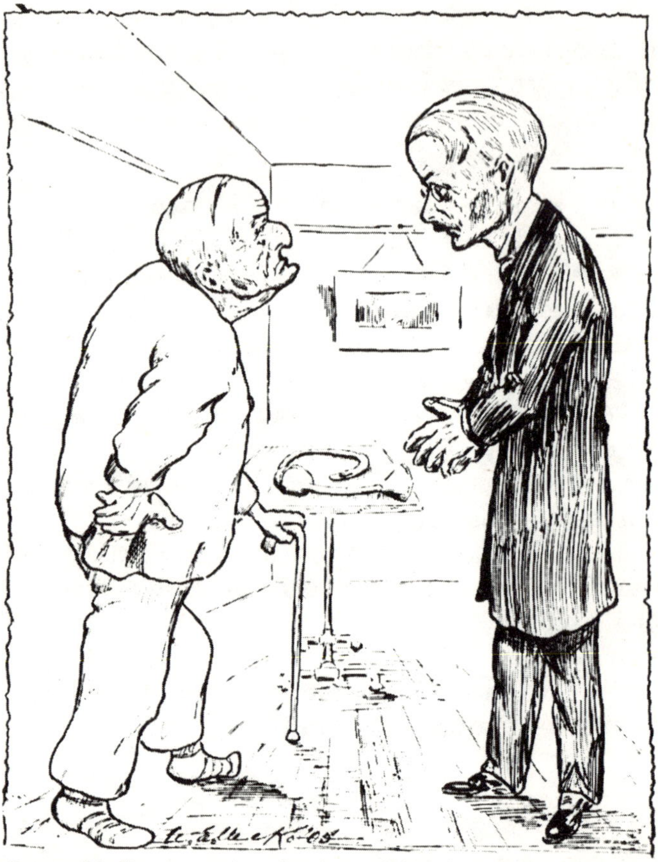

PROF. McP—D—N (to class): "There's nothing the matter with your back, sir. What you need is to have your stomach washed out."

Chapter Two

INTERNSHIP AND FIRST PRACTICE

AFTER GRADUATION CLARE proceeded to an internship at the Toronto General Hospital, a privilege he won as a result of competitive examinations. Nowadays in Canada, it is illegal to practise medicine without having served at least one year as intern in an approved hospital. This was not the case in 1907 when only a minority of graduates obtained this added education. Clare enjoyed the year, experiencing complete freedom of action for the first time in his life. Before this he had never lived away from home.

Among the physicians with whom he worked were Herbert Bruce, Perry Goldsmith, and Richard "Dicky" Reeve, the Dean. Bruce was a brilliant surgeon, but a man of rigid principles and beliefs who, as a consequence, provoked controversy. His later role as Inspector-General of the Canadian Army Medical Corps in World War I created much bitterness, his report on the Corps being very critical of the administrative structure. Although never fully implemented, most of the suggestions in his report were nonetheless adopted before the end of the war. Bruce later became Lieutenant-Governor of Ontario (1932-37).

Goldsmith was an eye, ear, nose, and throat specialist. On one occasion when he was to be out of the city for a few days, he entrusted a favourite patient to Clare's care. The patient was a woman with a mastoid infection that had led to the formation of a deep-seated brain abscess, and every day many yards of gauze dressing had to be removed from the abscess cavity and replaced with fresh gauze. So much gauze packing was required that it seemed enough to fill the entire skull, yet the patient remained quite stable and coherent. When presenting her at clinics to his medical students, Dr. Goldsmith would remark, out of earshot, how she demonstrated beyond doubt that women could get along as well without brains as with them. The remark would have drawn a hearty laugh eighty years ago.

Clare recalled another experience he had as an intern on the maternity service:

> One of my most interesting assignments at the hospital was in the Burnside section for obstetrics. One night when I was the only physician on call, five babies were born within a few minutes of each other. I sent for additional nurses who kept busy changing my gown and gloves for each delivery. All would have gone well had not Miss Snively, a distinguished previous Superintendent of Nurses, invented Snively Drawers for keeping the patients' legs warm during delivery. I was ready for a sterile gown. The nurse held up what we thought was a gown; I thrust my arms into the leg openings of the Snively Drawers. The sight was so ridiculous that we all burst into laughter ...

While at the Burnside, Clare and Dr. Kenneth McIlwraith delivered premature twins, who came to be known as "Kenny" and "Hincksie" after their medical attendants. The tiny creatures were displayed in an incubator in the medical exhibit at the Canadian National Exhibition.

Clare spent some time during his internship working on the service of Dr. Alexander McPhedran, the Professor of Medicine. McPhedran was an eloquent teacher, yet as a clinician he occasionally became enthusiastic over "fads" in diagnosis. During Clare's stay at the Toronto General Hospital a favourite diagnosis was "gastrosuccorhea," a label coined by Professor McPhedran. The prescribed treatment for such a condition involved stomach washing, an unpleasant procedure requiring the passage of a rubber tube through the mouth or nose into the stomach. The professor's patients viewed Clare with dismay as they saw him approach with the stomach tube in a basin of ice.

Clare recalled a distressing episode after he had decided that he needed experience in extracting teeth before venturing into private practice. He had never pulled a tooth, but he soon found an opportunity to do so when an elderly Irish lady was willing to have him remove a chronically aching tooth. A fellow intern, Dr. Fred Hamlin, similarly wanted experience in the use of the anaesthetic agent, nitrous oxide. The team was formed, instruments assembled, and the anaesthetic begun.

When the patient's face quickly turned blue, the anaesthetist became nervous. Clare hastily completed his first dental extraction. All seemed well until the patient, awakening from the anaesthetic, put her finger into her mouth and shouted at the top of her voice, "Why, he got the wrong tooth!" Clare hurriedly arranged to have a new tooth inserted at the Dental College to replace the one he had removed. By good fortune, this particular peccadillo never came to the attention of the hospital authorities.

He must have been a popular intern, at least with the nursing staff. After visiting a very ill patient late one night he stopped to have tea with a nurse. When the superintendent of nurses appeared at the end of the corridor, threatening to interrupt the forbidden fraternization, the nurse quickly turned down an empty bed and Clare crawled in, feigning sleep. To the relief of both conspirators, the incident went undiscovered.

As his year at the Toronto General came to an end, Clare learned of a job opportunity in Campbellford, Ontario, a small town in the vicinity of Peterborough and Belleville. A physician there asked him to look after his practice while he spent time in England preparing for the Fellowship of the Royal College of Surgeons. Clare accepted.

Before his departure from the hospital, the nursing staff presented Clare with a trunk full of obsolete obstetrical instruments, and as a gesture of mourning, graced his bedroom door with a woman's black stocking.

The name "Dr. C.M. Hincks" had no sooner appeared on a shingle in Campbellford than he was said to have performed a "miraculous" cure. While telling the story in later years Clare liked to quote from John Bunyan:

> Physicians get neither name nor fame by pricking of wheals or picking out thistles or by laying of plasters to the scratch of a pen; every old woman can do this. But if they would have a name and a fame, if they will have it quickly, they must, as I said, do some great and desperate cures. Let them fetch one to life that was dead; let them recover one to his wits that was mad; let them make one that was born blind to see, or let them give ripe wits to a fool; these are notable

> cures, and he that can do thus — if he doeth thus first he shall have the name and fame he deserves; he may lie a-bed till noon.[2]

One of Clare's first patients was the mayor of Campbellford. After hearing an account of the mayor's symptoms and completing an examination, he pronounced the diagnosis as paratyphoid fever. The disease closely resembles typhoid fever, with one significant difference: in those pre-antibiotic days paratyphoid fever lasted only about ten days, typhoid six to eight weeks. When the mayor returned to work within two weeks, recovered from what the townspeople thought was typhoid fever, all were amazed, and from that time forward Clare's waiting room in Campbellford was filled.

A short time after the mayor's recovery, Clare was credited with another impressive cure. Called to visit a young lad living in the country, he found the patient in a critical state from empyema, a disease in which pus forms in large quantities in the space between the chest wall and the lungs. The pus, on the left side, was under such pressure that it had pushed the heart towards the right side of the chest. The boy was desperately ill and emaciated. Informing the parents that their son would probably die if untreated, Clare indicated that the only chance lay in an immediate operation whereby an opening would have to be made through the chest wall to drain the pus. He advised the parents that, although the boy might not survive the operation, he should be removed at once to a hospital where he could be seen and treated by a surgeon.

In Clare's recollection, the boy's father responded: "Doctor, we want the operation done. We want you to do it, and we want it done right here in this farmhouse. If our boy is going to die, we want him to die in his own home."

> I was certainly on the spot. Surgery was not my forte. But, with the insistence of the boy's parents, there seemed to be no other course for me. Immediately I got in touch with Dr. Dick Bonneycastle, who was in Campbellford, and who had interned with me. I asked Dick if he would give the anaesthetic. He agreed, and added that he would bring along a new pair of rib cutters which he was anxious to try out.
>
> The boy was placed on the kitchen table, anaesthetized, and I began to work. The day was hot; I perspired. The incision I made was by no means straight. At last I got down to the ribs and stripped off the periosteum [the outer

covering of a rib]. The rib cutters worked wonderfully. An incision was made into the empyema cavity. At this, the pus, which had been under tremendous pressure, spurted out into the room; the heart, which had been crowded to the right, began to return to its proper position. Up to this time I had been a terrible surgeon, but the plight of my patient steadied my nerves. I placed a hand in the pleural cavity to slow the flow of pus.

However, the patient went into shock; heart action and breathing almost stopped. Bonneycastle administered strychnine and I started artificial respiration. The boy responded, and then I inserted a large drainage tube into the cavity, closed the wound and applied dressings. My patient made a remarkable recovery, gaining several pounds a week. The whole neighbourhood heard about it, and my waiting room became more crowded than ever.

Unfortunately, Clare's position as a bright young general practitioner in Campbellford was not to be sustained. The conflict between an ethical code that bound him and social pressure to break it, conspired to force him to leave the pleasant little town.

The difficulty began on an afternoon when Clare was visited by the mother of a young woman whom he had seen socially; he had been a dinner guest in the family's home. The lady stated that she was in the early stages of pregnancy. When Clare told her that he would be glad to provide care during her confinement, she replied that she wished to have the pregnancy terminated as soon as possible. Further, she informed him that the doctor whom he was replacing had done this for her frequently.

Clare could discover no medical justification for this or the previous abortions, which had been performed merely for her convenience. He told the lady he would give the matter serious consideration and would telephone his decision. Believing that abortion as contraception was ethically wrong, he declined to help her.

However, I did not want to continue living in a community with a family that had befriended me while I had to refuse to help one of its members. I got in touch with a lawyer to ascertain if my contract was binding with the doctor whose practice I was tending. He advised me that, since there was nothing in writing, the contract could be broken. And so, after notifying my patients, I left Campbellford after practising there for only three months and returned to Toronto.

Chapter Three

ESTABLISHING IN TORONTO

A SUCCESSFUL MEDICAL PRACTICE is not created merely by a decision to begin. Many factors contribute to success: location, willingness to work, good management, good luck and, above all, time to build goodwill. Clare was aware that a doctor can control only some of these factors; he quickly set out to find a suitable location for his new practice in Toronto.

Knowing that a young doctor without a good reputation would have difficulty in building up his practice, and that wherever he chose to practise he would be unknown, Clare approached the problem with cool calculation. He began to look for a house at the foot of a steep hill on the assumption that his office would be convenient for accident victims. Since automobiles were just coming into use and were not yet suited to winter conditions, tending to break down frequently, his reasoning was valid.

He rejected a house at the foot of the Avenue Road hill since the hill was so steep that the location might have more suitably employed an undertaker than a physician. Further south on Avenue Road, at Pears Avenue (just north of Davenport Road), there was a more gentle incline and it was there that Clare opened his first office in Toronto. He had predicted correctly; many of his first patients were indeed accident victims. Over time, however, most of his patients would come from families living in the immediate area.

Clare recorded an anecdote from his early days in Toronto that demonstrated his natural gift for handling people and their difficulties. When called to a home in the neighbourhood, he was greeted by several members of the family, all of whom were in tears:

> I asked if I was too late and was told: "Yes, Grandma has just passed on." I was taken to see Grandma, who was lying on a couch, her eyes closed, with members of the family standing around weeping. On feeling for Grandma's pulse, I found it was beating regularly and fairly strongly.
>
> I leaned over the elderly lady and whispered in her ear: "This is not St. Peter, but just a neighbour of yours here in Toronto. You will soon sit up and talk to your family. You are in good health."
>
> In a few minutes Grandma opened her eyes in an astonished way and looked around. The effect on the family was electric. They all felt they were witnessing a miracle.

Despite this evidence of his medical prowess, Clare's practice grew slowly. Forced to augment his modest income by becoming a demonstrator in biology at the University of Toronto, he occupied his time in the preparation and demonstration of specimens to teach embryology and the anatomy of the rabbit to students.

Life insurance examinations provided another source of income. Clare also acted as physician for Court McCaul of the Independent Order of Foresters, an organization in which his future father-in-law, Dr. Thomas Millman, was chief physician.

> Indeed, the very first dollar I made in Toronto was for a life insurance examination for the Foresters. I had this dollar framed and hung in my office. Unfortunately, I had to remove it later, when I got hard up and needed the dollar for current expenses.

It is an understatement to say that Clare was not well off at this point in his career. Besides conducting his own practice, he continued to work at the University, perform insurance examinations, and look after the practice of another Toronto doctor who was on extensive holidays — all to supplement his income. At the same time Clare became engaged to Mabel Millman, a young woman he had met at Windermere in his college days.

A brilliant student of modern languages, Mabel had received scholarships for postgraduate study at Bryn Mawr College in Pennsylvania as well as an institute in Spain, although she did not take advantage of the latter.

Clare expressed surprise, even many years later, that Mabel had selected him from her many suitors. The reason for her choice had little to do with any great material wealth that Clare could provide, since he was certainly unable to support a wife from the meagre earnings of his practice at Avenue Road. A short time later, when informed that a friend was leaving his practice on Dovercourt Road, Clare moved there in the hope of bettering his lot.

The move proved disastrous. Patients were few, and many could not have paid his bills had Clare even bothered to send them. One patient, however, took an interest in his affairs — a man by the name of Cowan who owned a drygoods store on Geary Avenue. One day he inquired if the practice was sufficiently busy. Clare lied, replying "Yes." On another occasion he asked the same question and received the same answer, but less emphatically. On a third questioning, Clare confessed that his practice was going badly.

Mr. Cowan responded that he had known all along how matters stood, the reason being, he said, that the office was not in the right location. He advised Clare to move the practice to his neighbourhood in "Shacktown" where he would find better business overnight. Clare followed this advice reluctantly, yet despite his misgivings his practice grew rapidly.

The change of fortune provided much personal and material gratification for Clare, yet, in spite of the improved circumstance, he later left his "shirt-sleeve" practice on Geary Avenue to move further north to St. Clair Avenue. Once again he was following the advice of his patient and neighbour, Mr. Cowan, who, observing the northward growth of Toronto, felt it would be advantageous for them both to follow the trend.

A suitable building was acquired at the corner of Dufferin Street and St. Clair Avenue. Although Clare leased the entire property he placed his office in the rear of the building. He was soon approached by a young graduate pharmacist by the name of R.E. Lapp who wished to establish a drug store on the corner site. After some initial hesitation Clare agreed and the "St. Clair Pharmacy" was the result.

The same Mr. Lapp later persuaded Clare to speculate in real estate. Lapp himself had hired another pharmacist to operate the drug store so that he could head a real estate venture, and when after only a few days in business he informed Clare that he had made $500 on a land deal, Clare was hooked. Although he had no plans to give up his practice, he thought it appeared easy to make a few extra dollars on the side. Approaching the real estate business with enthusiasm and ambition, he opened an office on Adelaide Street in Toronto's financial district, hired salesmen and, to complete the business image, purchased a large, expensive automobile.

For six months business went well, earning Clare $25,000. Inspired by his success, he decided he would reach $50,000 and then get out. The story is a familiar one. Just after reaching his $50,000 goal he lost $60,000 and, being an inexperienced businessman, he quit; instead of trying to recover his losses, Clare declared bankruptcy. It took him 10 years to repay the debt.

About the same time Clare had another expensive experience, this time involving mining stock. Some American promoters persuaded him to buy into what was, in retrospect, a distinctly shady operation. According to Clare's classmate, G.H. Gooderham, who had been brought into the "company," only Clare's appeal to philanthropist Joseph E. Atkinson saved the reputation of the pair, and perhaps kept them out of police records. Atkinson paid off their debts and the firm was dissolved.

> ... My financial reverse was a blessing in disguise. From this experience I discovered that in any venture, financial or otherwise, one should always be teamed up with able associates. I had been associated with other amateurs. I also learned in my hectic year what it is like to be a business man, and this knowledge helped me tremendously in dealing with financial men in Canada and the United States in subsequent years in connection with funding operations for mental health. Perhaps the most important lesson I learned was that to be stripped of every cent you have means very little to you in the long run. I made more friends when I was penniless than when I possessed a few dollars.

Clare's chronic state of financial misfortune led him to take another part-time position during his early days in Toronto. His appointment as District Medical Inspector for Schools in West Toronto was to have consequences of the utmost importance not only to Clare Hincks, but to the rest of Canada. The work proved to be the turning point in his professional life.

In his new position he had expected to meet children with the standard variety of physical ills, yet Clare soon discovered that was not the case. Although 60 percent of his school patients were in this category, with rashes, tonsillitis, malnutrition and other disorders, the remaining 40 percent had emotional, behavioural, and learning difficulties — problems which Clare, like most in his profession, was not qualified to deal with. Nothing he had been taught in medical school could guide him in the situations he faced.

All the disabilities that confronted Clare were mental–health related, although the term "mental health" did not exist at that time. No textbooks could provide the solutions he sought, for they were as yet unwritten. After an attempt to find some guidance at the University of Toronto, Clare was directed to a recently introduced course called Psychology.

> I enrolled in a graduate group composed of Professor W. G. Smith, E. J. Pratt, who developed into Canada's greatest poet, Ned Bott, who eventually headed the best Department of Psychology on the continent, and Helen McMurchie, who later married Ned Bott. We were a happy group, but I learned nothing about human nature and its operations.

There occurred in 1913 one of those fortunate events that bear results far beyond expectation. An announcement appeared in a Toronto newspaper of the Fourth International Congress of School Hygiene, to be held 25-30 August in Buffalo. In the hope that he would find someone at the conference would be able to help him, Clare decided to attend.

Transportation to Buffalo posed somewhat of a problem for Clare. Buffalo is over 100 miles from Toronto, and funds were still difficult to come by. So, once again, Hincks the doctor became Hincks the huckster who convinced John Bone, managing editor of the Toronto *Daily Star*, to hire him as a special reporter. With his expenses thus assured, Clare left for the Buffalo conference.

By good fortune, one of the conference speakers had worked with Binet and Simon in Paris during their development of intelligence testing. Alfred Binet, who had published his first plan for studying intelligence around 1895, had eventually collaborated with Simon, and the two men, working between 1905 and 1908, introduced a series of tests of graded difficulty which measured increasing degrees of mental ability or intelligence—the so-called IQ tests. Using these tests, it was considered possible to determine a person's mental age relative to his actual or chronological age. (The value of the test would later be questioned on the basis of limitations imposed by cultural conditioning, which pointed to the difficulty in using one test for all cultural groups. Yet, at the turn of the century, the test represented a major development in the still new field of psychology.) Simon and Binet's findings were originally published in French psychology journals between 1905 and 1908, and in a more extensive book format in 1911.

When Clare first heard of the Binet-Simon tests they were not in general use; in fact, to Clare's knowledge, they had not yet been used at all in Canada. After introducing himself to the visiting expert at the conference, Clare was generously provided training in the technique of administering the tests.

After his return to Toronto, he was eager to try out the new technique. However, thinking that West Toronto was probably not the place to begin, since the parents in his school district might object to their children being used in experiments, he was left with the question of where to find enough subjects. His dilemma was resolved when a friend, Judge Starr of the Toronto Juvenile Court, proposed that Clare test delinquents who appeared before the court. This he did for two years from an office at City Hall, during which time, having proved to his own satisfaction that the tests were reliable, he completed what appears to have been the first use of the tests in Canada.

Although it represented only one approach to the assessment of human personality and its functioning, intelligence testing became particularly important to Clare in his work in West Toronto schools, since mental retardation perplexed teachers more than any other problem at that time. Clare was able, through intelligence testing, to state fairly definitely whether a child's failure was due to basic inability, whatever the cause. Although factors other than intelligence had to be considered in the search for the reason for a child's failure or success, the degree of intellectual capacity was always significant.

As Clare's interest in children with mental deficiencies grew and his skill in using the Binet-Simon tests increased, he realized that he urgently needed a definite program of postgraduate training. He now knew in which field he wanted to specialize: psychiatry.

In those last days before World War I, the fashionable centre for psychiatric training was Vienna. But, for Clare, married, recently bankrupt and not yet profitably employed in his medical practice, Europe was out of the question. Fortunately, however, his work with intelligence testing had attracted the attention of Helen MacMurchy, another Toronto doctor who also was active in the field of mental deficiency (not to be confused with Helen McMurchie Bott, Clare's former co-student in psychology). She brought Clare's work to the attention of Dr. C.K. Clarke, who was then Dean of the Faculty of Medicine and Professor of Psychiatry at the University of Toronto, as well as Superintendent of the Toronto General Hospital — a person of power and influence in Canadian medicine.

Dr. Clarke met with Hincks and spoke of his desire to re-establish the out-patient psychiatric clinic at the Toronto General Hospital, the first of its kind in Canada. As Dr. Clarke relates:

> In 1909, when Superintendent of the Toronto Hospital for the Insane, I felt that something should be done to establish an Outdoor Clinic for psychiatric cases. It was only too evident that patients would be reluctant to seek help in a hospital for the insane, so permission was asked of the Board of Trustees of the [Toronto] General Hospital to establish a clinic in one of their buildings in the centre of the city. Dr. J.N.E. Brown, the Superintendent, approved of the scheme, interested the Trustees and obtained the necessary permission, placing at our disposal a room in what was known as the Ward Clinic, a little house on the corner of Chestnut and Christopher Streets. Dr. Ernest Jones, the well-known psychiatrist, who was at that time Associate Professor of Psychiatry, and also doing duty as Pathologist at the Toronto Hospital for the Insane, was assigned to the duty. This clinic did excellent work for a time in spite of the fact that it was difficult to make people understand its aims and intentions. With the building of the new General Hospital, the clinic house had to disappear, although it was maintained until the last moment possible. Dr. Jones returned to England, I assumed the Superintendency of the new General Hospital, and so great was the pressure of work that the thought of establishing a new clinic on a different basis was not entertained until Dr. Helen MacMurchy suggested that it should be resurrected, especially with the idea of helping the Juvenile Court to develop a special psychiatric study of many of its cases. At that date, Drs. C.M. Hincks and O.C.J. Withrow were endeavouring to assist in the examination of the court cases, but were working under great difficulties and without proper equipment. I was anxious to co-operate, consequently these young physicians came under our wing and transferred their energies to the newly formed clinic in April, 1914. [3]

Immediate success, attested by rapidly increased attendance, convinced even the sceptics of the usefulness of such a clinic. Yet sceptics did remain, and some, including physicians, laughed at what they called the "Nut Clinic."

As the clinic prospered, Hincks benefited from his association with Dr. Clarke. Regarded by Clare as the greatest psychiatrist Canada ever produced, Clarke had had 40 years of experience in the field, as Superintendent of the Rockwood Mental Hospital in Kingston, Ontario and later as Superintendent of the Provincial Mental Hospital in Toronto (famed as "999 Queen Street West"). Dr. Clarke loved mental patients as many people love children; his patients admired and cherished his empathetic nature and often remarked upon it. He was

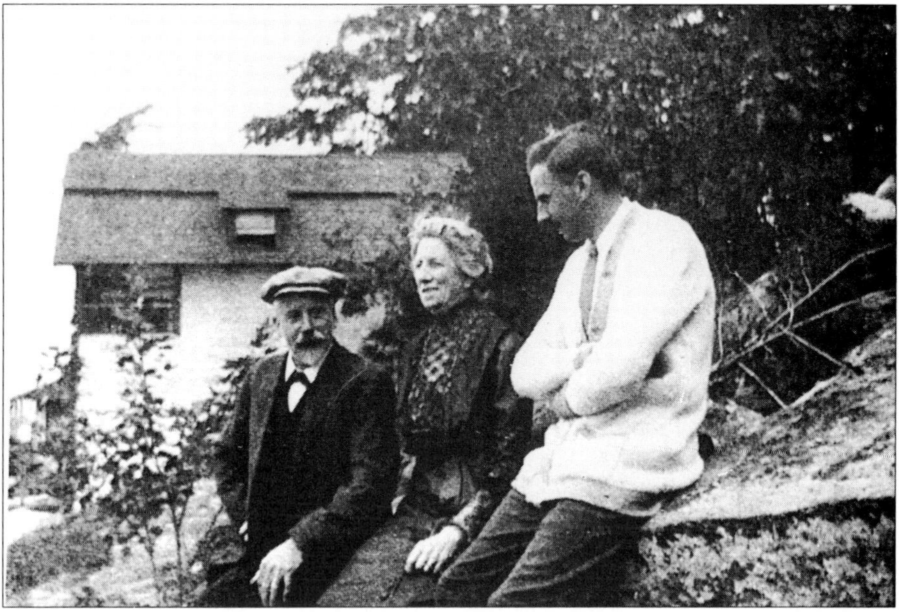

Clarence M. Hincks, with his parents at Windermere, Lake Rosseau, circa 1913 .

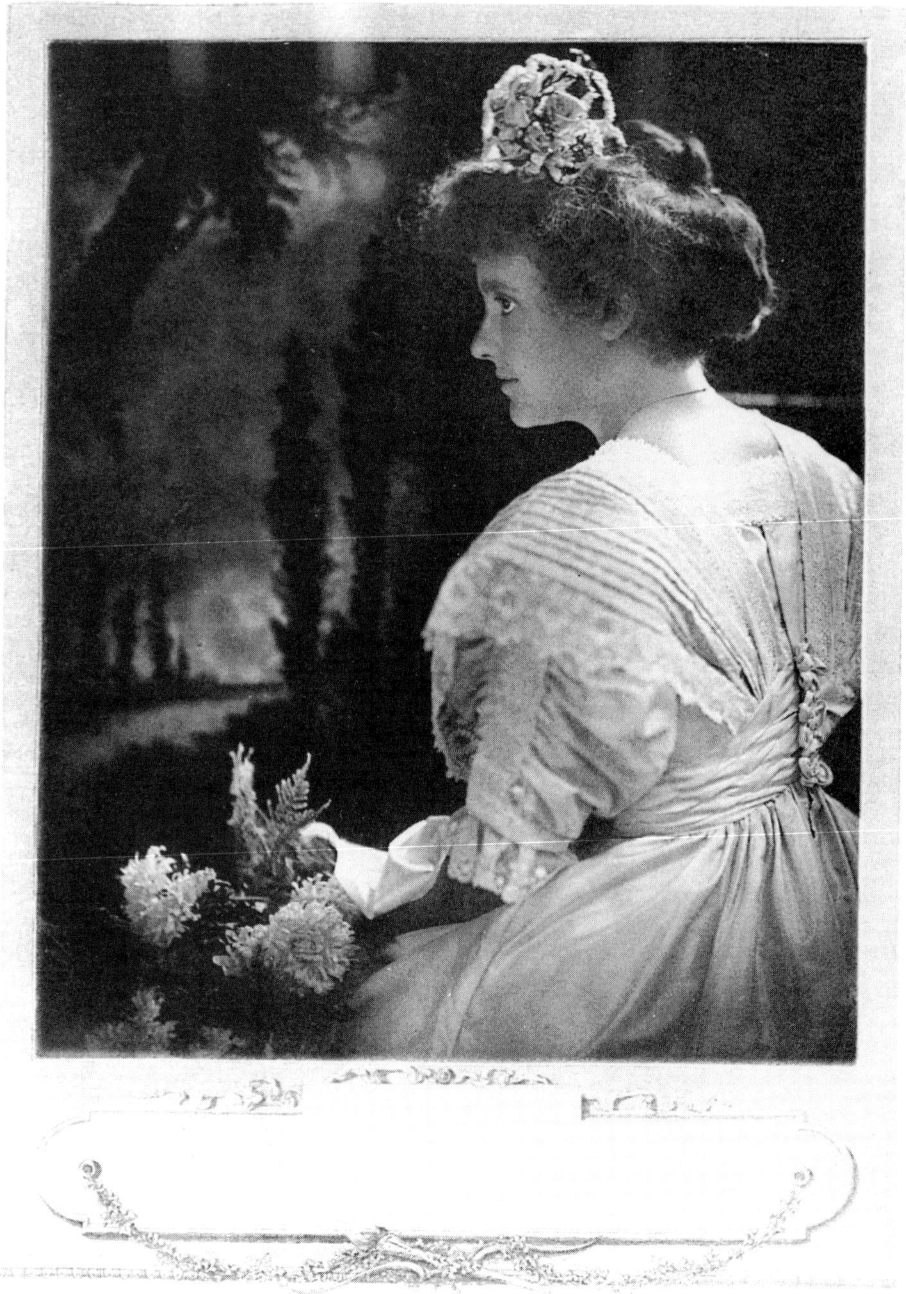

Mabel Helen Millman, shortly before her marriage to Clarence Meredith Hincks, 1912 .

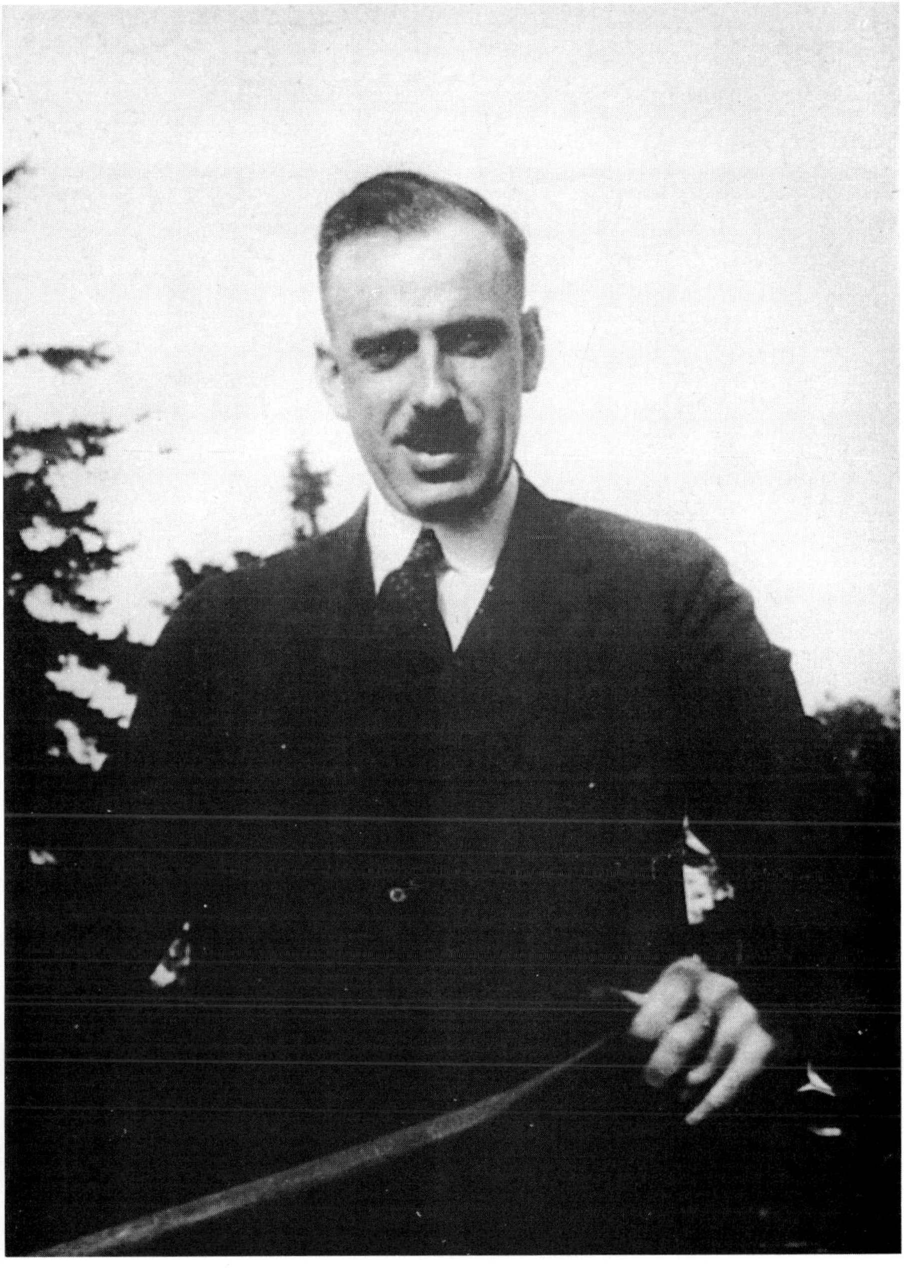

Clarence Meredith Hincks, on Lake Muskoka, circa 1923 .

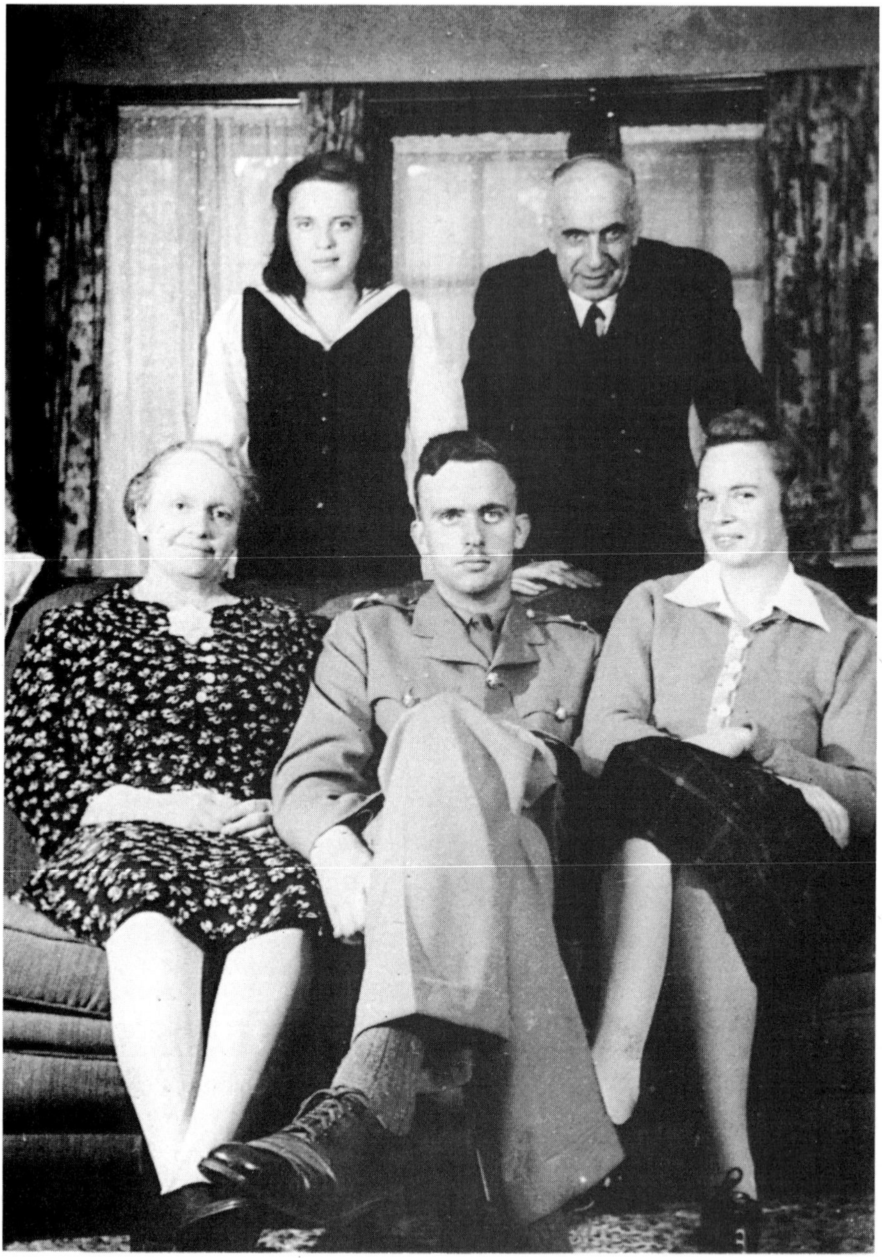

Back row: Barbara Hincks, Clarence Meredith Hincks; front row: Mabel Helen Hincks, William Hincks, and Margaret Hincks, June 1942.

a born psychiatrist and had the added advantage of a good European training. With his uncanny perception he could often diagnose a psychiatric condition in a matter of seconds. Consequently, he was an unusually successful clinician in the days before electroconvulsive therapy and modern anti-depressive drugs.

Clarke's affection for the mentally ill was quite genuine. After leaving 999 Queen Street and finding life lonely without his patients, he always had a housemaid in his home who suffered from delusions or some other form of mental illness. Perhaps some of Clarke's interest in Hincks's work stemmed from his understanding of Clare's sympathy for his juvenile patients.

> And so, Dr. Clarke became my father in psychiatry and was the guiding influence for Dr. Withrow, Marjorie Keyes and myself. My specialist training was now assured, and it was the very best training possible because I was apprenticed to a great man.

Miss E. De V. Clarke, Dr. Clarke's daughter, had been appointed social worker at the clinic. As a graduate in nursing from New York Presbyterian Hospital she had considerable experience with cases of mental disease and defect. When, during the war, No. 4 Canadian General Hospital was organized, Miss Clarke enlisted and went overseas with it, leaving the social work to Miss Marjorie Keyes, a student nurse training in the psychiatric clinic who would remain with the clinic staff after graduation.

Dr. Withrow had also left the clinic during the war years to serve overseas. He never returned to mental hygiene work, although he maintained a vigorous interest in matters of social welfare and social progress in general. Withrow achieved considerable notoriety in the 1920s when he was convicted and imprisoned for performing an illegal abortion, a charge he denied strenuously. After release from Kingston Penitentiary he launched an attack on the indifference of officials to the brutal treatment of Canadian prison inmates, and published a book on the subject. Hincks and Withrow had maintained their friendship through this time; Clare later wrote the preface to Withrow's book, *Unshackling the Transgressors*.

Clare did not enlist in the armed forces during the First World War, partly due to Dr. Clarke's advice to remain in Toronto where he could continue his work with the mentally ill. The Canadian Army Medical Corps offered no psychiatric service, and no special screening procedure for the recognition of psychosis or neurosis in enlisted men was carried out at the time of induction.

The out-patient psychiatric clinic at the Toronto General Hospital continued to enjoy remarkable success, with attendance increasing steadily. Patients attended at their own instigation, some with relatives or friends, and others were referred by a variety of government and social service agencies. The clinic provided help to hundreds, sometimes preventing suicide, and often giving its patients a new start in life.

Besides assisting the mentally ill, the clinic also served to educate many physicians, nurses, and social workers entering the complex field of mental hygiene. Visitors from other centres came to study the clinic and the concept behind it and, possibly most important, a great public educational process began, a program to which Clare Hincks would devote his life. "Normal" people had begun to realize that the mentally ill were not as completely and irrevocably abnormal as had been believed; nor were they, the normal, as normal as they had thought. The twin concepts of gradations of normality and of the curability of many forms of mental disability, were advocated constantly by Hincks, Withrow and the clinic staff.

Even recently these concepts had still not found universal acceptance. Dr. Karl Menninger, in a lecture to a lay audience in 1958, reiterated the same ideas:

> ... mental illness is something that may occur in the lives of any of us. It always develops rather unexpectedly .... I do not want you to be alarmed by this statement. But I do want to break through the barrier of misapprehensions that divides the world into "those people" meaning this time those impossible, out-landish, afflicted "crazy" people — and "us" — us sane, sensible people. That is the perfectly understandable, aristocratic view, but it is a mistaken one .... The general notion has long prevailed that, once mental illness has appeared, the victim is doomed .... This all seems incredible to us today, because we have quite the opposite view. Most attacks of mental illness subside; most of the patients recover.[4]

Recognizing that the accomplishments at the clinic were only a beginning, Clare knew that much more had to be done. Mental hygiene training had to be introduced throughout the country; the asylums had to be assessed and reorganized, since facilities for the mentally ill appeared to be inadequate in every way; psychiatric screening for immigrants was urgently required, and much research was needed. The work at the clinic merely indicated the magnitude of the problem at hand.

Chapter Four

THE CANADIAN NATIONAL COMMITTEE FOR MENTAL HYGIENE

AFTER TWO YEARS at the clinic Clare confided to Dr. Clarke his ambitions for the future of mental health. Clarke was sympathetic and encouraged his young associate to explore further the wide field of psychiatry. Since few options were available at that time in Canada, Clare decided to visit New York, the centre of psychiatric training in North America. By the time of his return he would have established a framework for his dream of a better deal for the mentally handicapped in Canada. In New York he discovered Clifford Beers and the mental hygiene movement.

Clare's momentous trip was made in the autumn of 1917. His first day in New York was spent calling on psychiatrists, most of whom, after listening to Clare's recital of inadequacies in Canada, were barren of useful advice, although one man suggested that he meet with a group called the National Committee for Mental Hygiene. There he spoke with the Associate Medical Director, Dr. Frankwood Williams, a pleasant man who was sympathetic to his plight, yet still unable to offer any helpful suggestions. Thanking him, Clare prepared to leave.

On his way out Clare met a young employee, Mr. Paul Komora, who asked if he was leaving without meeting the Secretary of the National Committee and the founder of the mental hygiene movement, Mr. Clifford Beers.

> Although I had never heard of Mr. Beers, I told Mr. Komora that I would be glad to chat with him. When I met Mr. Beers, I told him what I was looking for. He said: "You have come to the right place, but have you read my book, *A Mind that Found Itself*? When I replied in the negative, he handed me a copy and asked me to read it that night and return to see him the following morning. When I told Mr. Beers that I had never in my life read an entire book at one sitting, he assured me that I would read this one. He was right. I finished it at three o'clock in the morning.

Beers had actually been a delegate at the Buffalo conference of 1913, and a laudatory account of him and his book appeared in one of Clare's news reports in the *Toronto Star* on 26 August 1913. Of course, Clare's autobiographical notes, in which the above quotation appears, were not prepared until 1962, so it is not surprising that errors occurred in names and temporal relationships. Certainly Beer's influence on Clare didn't begin until 1918.

In *A Mind that Found Itself*, Beers relates his two-year experience as a patient in public and private mental institutions in Connecticut. Clifford Whittingham Beers (1878?-1943) had graduated from the Sheffield School of Engineering at Yale and just after graduation had become severely depressed. In a suicide attempt he jumped from a third-storey window of his home and broke his legs. He was immediately placed in a private hospital and later transferred to a public institution, yet in each place his treatment lacked understanding and was at times brutal. Fortunately, he recovered despite the quality of treatment.

In convalescence Beers wrote the book which recorded his feelings and experiences during more than two years of hospitalization. As one can imagine, it was difficult 60 years ago for a former inmate of a "lunatic asylum" to have a book published at all. Fortunately for Beers, William James, the noted philosopher, read the manuscript and pronounced it a classic. He then wrote the introduction to the first edition.

A Mind That Found Itself was a success, with profits from its sale being used to launch what Beers called the Mental Hygiene Movement, and establishing in Connecticut in 1908 the first Mental Hygiene Society in the world. This venture was so successful that in 1909 he created a national organization which, in turn, prospered. Beers surrounded himself with able medical scientists, and he appeared to have the Midas touch for raising large sums of money for the work in hand.

Clare finished reading Beers' book in the middle of the night, and when the two men met on the following day Clare expressed his strong interest in the mental hygiene work being done in New York, indicating that the same was needed in Canada. Beers' enthusiasm reflected his ambition to make the movement an international one, and thus Clare was able to persuade Beers to speak in Canada on the subject of mental hygiene as soon as an organization could be established.

Having found the assistance and encouragement he'd been seeking, Clare returned to Canada. He did not, however, begin organizing in Toronto, but in Montreal. Recognizing that success depended on his ability to obtain the blessing of a substantial portion of the medical profession, he thought he was more likely to receive a sympathetic hearing in Montreal where he was unknown, than in Toronto where he was known to be a general practitioner of no particular consequence except that he had dabbled in mental health under Clarke's guidance.

Clare had previously met Dr. Colin K. Russel (1877-1956), a well-known neurologist in Montreal who was serving as consulting neuropsychiatrist to the Canadian army, and who was well aware of problems created by enlisting men who were mentally ill. Since Russel was also Lecturer in Clinical Neurology at McGill University, Clare thought he might be in a position to arrange a meeting for him with the Faculty of Medicine. Dr. Russel happened to be out of town, but his associate, Dr. Gordon Mundie, offered to invite all members of the medical faculty to meet at the University Club:

> I was quite unknown in Montreal and I wondered if any medical men would turn up. To my amazement Sir William Peterson, the Principal of McGill University and the entire medical faculty were on hand. Later I was told that McGill was smarting because some of its distinguished staff members had been lured to the University of Toronto. When it was learned that I was from Toronto suspicion was aroused, and it was felt that Toronto might be using a new tactic by sending an unknown. Staff members were ready to put a stop to it; and so they all turned up.

Whatever their reason for attending, Clare had his audience. He spoke to them of the deficiencies in Canadian training and of the lack of facilities for assisting the mentally ill. He outlined the activities of the Psychiatric Clinic in Toronto, as well as the major conclusion derived from its experience — that serious mental disability was widespread and that a strong national organization was needed to conduct surveys, to promote better training of personnel and to encourage research. He also told the story of Clifford Beers, and added that his help was available if requested.

The scheme was discussed by those present, and Sir William Peterson, lending the weight of his authority, remarked that a national mental hygiene organization was long overdue, and promised full support for the plan. Dr. Hincks was asked to call on them again and to keep the faculty informed of future developments.

Clare's next move was to Ottawa, where he called on the Governor-General, the Duke of Devonshire, and was received at Rideau Hall with great courtesy and affability. After hearing the Duke's admonition not to use medical jargon because "I would not understand you. You know, I am a farmer," Clare repeated his story of problems and solutions, deficiencies and ignorance. At that point in the war, recruits who did not even know who the enemy was were joining the Canadian army. Some, Clare said, because of grossly low mentality, were as likely to shoot their own men as the enemy. Other cases existed where, because of a shortage of hospital beds, many mental patients were in jails even though they had committed no offence. Clare's graphic recitation of the Canadian situation impressed the Duke, and when he reported that the medical faculty at McGill University backed him in his aims, the Duke's interest was evident; he asked what was required of him to further this work. Clare said that the Duke's interest and sponsorship in developing a national organization would be extremely important.

> The Governor-General replied, "All right, I will be pleased to give my patronage when your board requests me to do so." "But," I said, "we have no board." The Duke was perplexed: "You want my patronage for something that does not exist?" I replied that that was exactly what we wanted. A national organization in our field could not possibly succeed unless we had a Board composed of top leaders in Canada—men who were known to all Canadians and who were respected by them. I explained that if he would endorse us now, I would use his name and be in a position to assemble the strongest board in Canada. The Governor-General thought a minute and then said: "You win. I will extend my patronage now, even though I am acting contrary to all precedents. My wife will help you also."

Two major hurdles had thus been cleared on the road to forming a national mental health organization. The medical faculty of an important Canadian university backed the scheme, and the Governor-General's patronage was promised. Clare then returned to Montreal and met with Sir William Peterson, who supplied him with a list of 20 distinguished Canadians suitable for the Board of Directors of the as yet unnamed organization. Clare called on all of these men, and 18 of the 20 agreed to act. Among them were Lord Shaughnessy, President of the Canadian Pacific Railway; Mr. E. W. Beatty (later Sir Edward), Vice-President of the C.P.R.; Mr. R. B. Angus, one of the three builders of the C.P.R.; Dr. Charles F. Martin, Professor of Medicine, McGill University; Sir Vincent Meredith, President of the Bank of Montreal; Sir George Burn, President of the Bank of Ottawa; Sir William Price, of the Price Brothers lumber empire; Mr. F.W. Molson, President of Molson's Brewery; Mr. D.A. Dunlap, Secretary-Treasurer of Hollinger Gold Mine; Vincent Massey; and Mr. John B. Holden, chief legal counsel for the Hollinger interests. These men, along with Professor Ned Pratt of the University of Toronto, accompanied Clare back to Ottawa and, with the Duke of Devonshire chairing the proceedings, the Canadian National Committee for Mental Hygiene (later the Canadian Mental Health Association) was formally and legally instituted on 26 April 1918. The total time required to carry out this feat of organization, of progressing from a vision to a national committee with vice-regal patronage, was just a few weeks.

Having completed the legal formalities, Clare turned to the task of raising money for the initial work of the new organization. He tells how this was arranged:

> Toward this end, I secured the co-operation of three hostesses — one each in Toronto, Quebec City, and Montreal. Each of these hostesses would give a tea in her home, to which twenty guests would be invited to meet Clifford Beers and me. The first of these teas was held in the home of Mr. and Mrs. D.A. Dunlap, of Toronto. I introduced Clifford Beers, who told the dramatic story of his life. Neither one of us asked for money, but at the conclusion of Beers' talk, Mrs. H.D. Warren, one of the guests and at the time the First Lady of Toronto, approached me and asked if we needed money. I said we did, and she replied that no one in the room would ever feel more like giving than right then. With this prompting I handed a piece of paper and a

> pencil to Mrs. Warren. She signed her name, pledging $3,000, and said: "If I am wrong in my guess that the others present will contribute, then I will raise my subscription to $15,000." The paper was then passed around and $24,000 was raised in less than three minutes. Beers and I repeated the performance in Quebec City and Montreal with similar financial success.

With the drafting of a formal organization and the opening of a bank account, an office, an executive, and a staff were required to begin the real work of the Committee. An office was rented near the Toronto General Hospital, and the Board elected Dr. Charles F. Martin (1868-1953) as President, Sir Edward W. Beatty as Chairman of the Board, Dr. C.K. Clarke as Medical Director, Miss Marjorie Keyes as Social Worker, and Dr. Hincks as Associate Medical Director and Secretary.

Chapter Five

ASPIRATIONS AND ACCOMPLISHMENTS

CONCRETE ACHIEVEMENT WAS now required to justify the existence of the newly established Canadian National Committee for Mental Hygiene. As it happened, an urgent problem, very much in the Committee's range of interest, arose for consideration when Dr. C.K. Russel who was in charge of neuropsychiatry for the Canadian army, inspected all hospitals in Canada that were treating military cases. When Russel visited Manitoba and discovered that treatment facilities there were inadequate, he proposed to remove military patients to other centres. The government was dismayed, assuming that if its asylums were unsuitable for soldiers they must also be unsuitable for civilians. Appealing to Russel for advice, it was told that the Canadian National Committee for Mental Hygiene had just been organized and would be prepared to survey the public facilities in Manitoba. Further, if the government would implement the recommendations arising from the study, the military patients would be left in Manitoba.

The provincial government acted quickly, and in July, 1918, Russel, in his role as Chairman of the Executive Committee of the CNCMH, received a letter from the Public Welfare Commission of Manitoba asking the Committee to make a study of mental health conditions in that province. The Commission, formed a year earlier in 1917, included among its members A.T. Mathers, MD, a prominent psychiatrist, and Mrs. J. Halpenny, the wife of Jasper Halpenny, MD, also a psychiatrist. The surveyors began work at the beginning of October.

In an introduction to the official report of the survey, details of the government's initial request were outlined:

> In July, 1918 Lieut.-Colonel Colin K. Russel, Chairman of the Executive of the Canadian National Committee for Mental Hygiene, received a letter from the Public Welfare Commission of the Province of Manitoba, requesting the National Committee to make a study of social conditions in that province, with special reference to the insane and feeble-minded. It was indicated that the Committee would be given a free hand in connection with the survey, and that every facility would be placed at its disposal for the purpose. The Executive [of the Canadian National Committee], when assured that the study would be undertaken with the full sanction and approval of the Manitoba Government, instructed the Medical Director, Associate Medical Director, and Social Worker, to visit Manitoba and begin the work immediately. Some time was lost in completing arrangements, but early in October the survey was commenced and pursued diligently until finished. [5]

The Committee was to study the province's two hospitals for the insane at Brandon and Selkirk, as well as jails, general hospitals, and a variety of homes and other institutions in Manitoba. The findings of the survey were astonishing; it is difficult for today's reader to believe that the account of conditions in the asylums was not taken from an earlier century.

In its first stages, the survey was conducted by Doctor Hincks and Miss Marjorie Keyes, although Doctor Clarke later joined them in Winnipeg. Visiting many institutions between the first and the eighteenth of October, they spent almost three weeks in the province.

How bad were conditions in 1918? And were they worse in Manitoba than in other provinces? Many patients in Manitoba's public and private institutions were certainly not well treated by modern psychiatric standards, although it would soon become evident that other provinces were experiencing problems of equal urgency.

Clare and Miss Keyes spent the first few days of their visit in Winnipeg assessing a number of institutions there. Beginning with the Salvation Army Industrial Home, they proceeded to the Juvenile

Court, several public schools, and the Home of the Good Shepherd. Although they encountered situations worthy of criticism, their findings were neither startling nor unexpected. In the following week, however, they visited the Home for Incurables in Portage la Prairie, where they found conditions so bad that they immediately returned to Winnipeg to consult with government officials. At the same time they wired Clarke to ask him to join the inspection party as quickly as possible. Both Clare and Miss Keyes had already seen many asylums and similar institutions, so what had they found so upsetting at the Portage home? In the words of the confidential report submitted to Mr. Norris's government, and signed by Clarke and Hincks:

> The most painful and distressing survey undertaken while we were in Manitoba was at the so-called Home for Incurables at Portage la Prairie. Two visits were made, the first on October 8, 1918, the second on October 15, 1918, as we did not wish to labour under any misapprehension in regard to what was seen there. The name, Home for Incurables, is misleading, and the institution has become a recuperation house for every kind of ailment, — as one of our party expressed it, "from eczema to dementia." Apparently any family in Manitoba which had a troublesome member, either old or young, sent them here, until this institution possessed an unhappy conglomeration of idiots, imbeciles, epileptics, insane, seniles, and mentally normal people suffering from incurable diseases. Of course, this state of affairs is the outcome of the want of proper institutions in the province to care for the different classes represented, but it is difficult to realize the system of inspection which allowed such a condition of affairs to develop. That insane people should be housed in this institution is astonishing, as it is devoid of any equipment for caring for cases of insanity. The result has been tragic in the extreme, and we may well pass by most of the details of what might be the unpleasant task of describing what we saw, knowing that the government will take immediate steps to put an end to the abuses existing, as soon as they are brought to the attention of the Attorney General.

One of the reasons for the unhappy state of affairs at the Home for Incurables was the name of the institution. At that time, the stigma of having a relative incarcerated in an "asylum" or a "hospital for the insane" was insufferable, yet if families could declare to the world that one of their members was in a home for incurables, they were more likely to receive sympathy than ostracism.

The superintendent of the home at Portage la Prairie, although an efficient housekeeper, was totally untrained in the medical or nursing care of any of her patients. The physician who visited the home daily was also without psychiatric training, and admitted to Clare that he did not attempt to make diagnoses but accepted the statement of the referring physician. Theoretically, no insane patients were allowed admission to the home, but in fact many were present. Of 335 patients in residence when the inspection was carried out, 102 were classified as "feebleminded," "imbecile," or "idiot." No occupation whatever was provided for their diversion during incarceration, so the patients simply existed there until death brought merciful release.

Overcrowding was a serious problem at the Portage la Prairie home. Three hundred and thirty-five patients were accommodated in a space designed for about 200. One room, measuring 18 by 8 feet, contained 16 beds — which must have been bunk beds in order to fit into such a tiny space. Further, the report indicated that the ventilation of the home, at best, was not good — a bald remark that nevertheless speaks volumes to anyone familiar with this type of institution.

Inmates were often physically restrained and held in seclusion at the Home for Incurables. The inspectors counted six patients in muffs, a device used for tying together and wrapping the hands in canvas to prevent violence or destruction. To the question "What are you going to do with such unmanageable creatures?" the report emphatically replied that these "creatures" would never have sunk to the level they did had they been cared for intelligently in the early stages of their disease.

The rooms used for seclusion within the home were actually cells, without light or ventilation, and Clare warned that they should be eliminated at once. At the end of a long dark ward a closet was found containing a naked woman with deathly pale skin. The tiny space contained no furniture, no bed, not even a mattress, and when the door was opened the woman placed a small fragment of shawl over her eyes, obviously unaccustomed to light. When asked how long this woman had been in the closet, the Superintendent replied, "Two years." Clare asked how often she had been permitted out during that period. "Once, and then only for ten minutes in a cage. She was restless, so we returned her to the cupboard."

Lack of professional care, overcrowding, public indifference or revulsion, inadequate facilities, and sometimes cruel, archaic treatment were all too apparent at the Home for Incurables.

Following the first visit to Portage, Clare and Miss Keyes inspected the Winnipeg, Portage la Prairie, and Brandon jails. Manitoba law in 1918 required that every patient sent to a mental asylum be committed by a magistrate; voluntary commitment was not permitted. Most committed mental patients had therefore been jailed for at least a brief period, sent by a magistrate to await transfer to the "appropriate" institution as space became available or, one suspects, at the whim of officialdom.

Aside from the unfavourable effect of such indignity and humiliation on disturbed minds, the victims of this unhappy system were exposed to additional hazards. The treatment administered in jail was not at all of a trained psychiatric nature, although a patient who became violent or abusive could expect attention. Patients often arrived at the asylum battered and bruised, and the actual transfer was sometimes effected by chaining the patient to a metal grill for easy handling.

It is typical of the reports submitted by the Committee to Manitoba and other provinces — and particularly typical of both Clarke and Hincks — that, while not hesitating to expose the inadequacies and abuses, they rarely blamed the individuals responsible for them. Thus, in appraising the jail system, the report concluded:

> Much as we deprecate the conditions as found, we realize that it is scarcely fair to censure the officials who have a task imposed on them which they are not trained to undertake. They simply do their best to meet an awkward situation.

A similar attitude invested the comments written after inspection of the Brandon Hospital for the Insane. Clare was keenly aware of deficiencies in that particular asylum, yet he was quick to point out that the Medical Superintendent, J.B. Chambers, MD, was the only physician to care for 700 patients, and simply could not be expected to do much more than attend to the innumerable demands of administration. Clare, in his unpublished autobiographical notes, described his first impressions of the Brandon institution:

> I will never forget the shock I received when we started our study at the Brandon Asylum. There were 700 patients with only one physician, who was the superintendent. Practi-

> cally all his time was spent in supervising the asylum farm and in filling in death certificates. He had no time for the treatment of patients. There was not one trained nurse in the establishment. The male attendants were the roughest looking group of men I had ever seen. They walked about without collars and presented a dishevelled appearance. Because of the number of black eyes among the patients, it was evident that these attendants used strong arm methods for control. Over many of the beds there had been placed heavy iron grating giving the patients underneath the appearance of caged wild animals. Patients sat in complete idleness on long hard wooden benches, many of them in physical restraint, staring vacantly into space, dejected, waiting for death to give them release. Restless patients were placed in solitary confinement in small desolate rooms.

Such was the situation in Manitoba as recently as 1918; the origins of such treatment are found in the instructions given by Dr. John Haslam in a book published in 1809:

> ... the patient should be kept alone in a dark and quiet room, so that he may not be affected by the stimuli of light or sound .... The hands should be properly secured, and the patient should also be confined by one leg; this will prevent him from committing any violence. The more effectual and convenient mode of confining the hands is by metallic manacles; for, should the patient, as frequently occurs, be constantly endeavouring to liberate himself, the friction of the skin sustained without injury [will restrain him] .... The straight waistcoat is admirably calculated to prevent patients from doing mischief to themselves.

Although it would seem that improvement in the treatment of mental illness in Manitoba was a long way off, the province had in fact already begun plans for the first psychopathic hospital in Canada even before the Committee began its survey. The establishment of such an institution was a project that Clarke had been recommending in Ontario for many years, and as he and Clare reviewed the architect's plans during their stay in Winnipeg, Clarke must have felt some degree of envy mixed with the pride of seeing his proselytizing take root in a province other than his own.

In the official report, however, opinion about the psychopathic hospital was decidedly guarded, with Clarke and Hincks emphasizing that the building of such a hospital did not remove the need for improvements at Selkirk and Brandon. Since only 25 beds had been planned for the new hospital, the report suggested that it might become simply a reception centre of limited capacity, a prediction that proved largely accurate.

Inspection of the Selkirk Hospital for the Insane brought the survey near to a close. The findings there were similar to those at Brandon and many of the other institutions visited — a staff that was grossly deficient in numbers and training, and, as at Brandon, a single resident physician who was required to care for up to 400 patients and carry all the responsibilities of administration. No trained nurses were employed although 34 male and 25 female attendants made up the "nursing staff," functioning, it must be assumed, as custodians. No attempt was made to keep accurate or complete records of cases, thus no basis for research existed, nor were any laboratory facilities available.

The Committee concluded the section of the report dealing with the Selkirk Hospital:

> Selkirk is on the whole admirably managed as a custodial institution, but totally unfitted to meet the modern demands of a hospital for the insane of advanced type. The management was to be heartily congratulated on having achieved such excellent results with such meagre equipment and resources.

Appalled by the conditions in general they found in Manitoba, the Committee members responded explicitly and forcefully to the provincial authorities:

> The hospitals for the insane in Manitoba are organized without the slightest regard to the demands of modern science; they have neither staff nor equipment to make them anything more than custodial institutions, and proper medical treatment is not provided .... We use the word "asylums" here, advisedly, as the majority of these institutions cannot by any stretch of imagination be called hospitals.

The confidential report of the Committee to the Public Welfare Commission included a number of recommendations for action. It is instructive now to see how closely they were followed after the Welfare Commission in turn prepared and submitted its recommendations to the Manitoba government. A few excerpts from the Commission's report will indicate how much this group actually depended on the findings of the Canadian National Committee:

> Hospitals for the Insane should be regarded as being on the same plane as other hospitals and no longer as mere custodial institutions ....
>
> Hospitals for the insane in Manitoba are at present organized without regard to the demands of modern science. They have neither adequate staff nor equipment to make them anything more than custodial institutions. While the Winnipeg General Hospital, for example, has seventy-two attending physicians and surgeons, and eighteen internes in addition to that of the Laboratory and Pathological Departments, the Brandon Hospital for the Insane, of approximately the same size, has only one physician. His duties are practically all administrative ....
>
> ... diagnosis of all supposed cases of insanity should in future be made by competent Psychiatrists, either at the Psychopathic department of the Winnipeg General Hospital or at the reception department which is recommended as an addition to the Hospital for the Insane at Brandon. Commitment from these reception departments to the Insane Hospitals should be made direct, and not as at present by a Magistrate through the gaols.
>
> In this connection we must express regret that the new Psychopathic Ward, now being erected at the Winnipeg General Hospital, is not of sufficient size to meet the requirements ....
>
> ... the most important requirement follows after, and that is the employment of capable and efficient people for the conduct of the work in these various institutions. Personnel is the important factor. Too much stress cannot be laid upon the requirements of character and training of those in charge of the people of these classes. Not only must those in charge be capable, but their assistants must understand the dignity and importance of their work. To insure continuity of efficient services, competent training, special education, and suitable remuneration with proper living quarters should be provided for those to whom the Province commits the destinies of its most unfortunate and afflicted citizens.

Some suggestions were not acted upon by the Manitoba government. The Committee report had recommended segregating the "chronic insane" at Brandon Hospital, and the mentally retarded at Selkirk, yet neither change appeared to have been made, even though this recommendation was included in the Public Welfare Commission's report to the government in 1919.

The first session of the Manitoba Legislature after receipt of the Commission's Report opened on 23 January 1919. The Speech from the Throne

> ... mentioned the work of the Public Welfare Commission, its survey and the special classification of mental diseases and the near ... completion of the Psychopathic Institute which, as part of the Winnipeg General Hospital, would introduce into the new system of treatment the most humane and scientific methods anywhere in vogue and prevent mental cases from passing through the gaols as in the past.

The Canadian National Committee for Mental Hygiene was not mentioned in the throne speech. Clare emphasized in his autobiographical notes that as long as the Committee conducted surveys, it adhered to the policy of reporting to the government alone and not releasing reports to the press or other bodies; the organization chose to remain in the background, not seeking to advance the name of the Committee but preferring a reputation for close co-operation with the source of power and reform — government. In recent years the Canadian Mental Health Association has changed this policy, becoming an organization with large public membership and attendant publicity around fund-raising drives and other campaigns. The Association continues its co-operation with government, but the route of pressure on government has changed to greater reliance on public participation and responsibility.

Elimination of the archaic system of committing patients through the jails was one reform that the Committee emphasized in its report. Later in the January session, the Honorable Dr. R.S. Thornton, Minister of Education, himself a physician, introduced a bill regarding the treatment of mentally diseased patients. The bill provided that such patients be sent directly to the Psychopathic Hospital instead of appearing before a magistrate for committal, a measure that was passed under the Mental Diseases Act of 1919. This Act provided for other matters of mental health such as the change of name from "Insane Hospital" to "Hospital for Mental Diseases" and for the voluntary commitment of patients to these and other facilities. While it appears that detention in a jail was still not prohibited, it no longer remained the standard practice. The legislation reads:

> ... the justice or justices may thereupon by his or their warrant commit such person to the custody of the constable or other person who apprehended him or to such safe custody as the justice or justices may deem fit, and shall order the person so apprehended to be conveyed as soon as convenient to the psychopathic ward, or to one of the said hospitals.

The Mental Diseases Act further provided that the Lieutenant-Governor in Council be authorized to forge rules and regulations for the management and internal economy of the psychopathic ward in each hospital, as well as for the conduct of the officers, employees, and patients therein. Physical abuse of patients was specifically prohibited, and penalties were provided for those found using such barbaric treatment methods.

What factors have contributed to the radical improvement in Manitoba's care of the mentally ill since the Committee's work there in 1918? The first, and unquestionably the most decisive factor has been a change in public and professional attitudes towards the plight of the mentally ill.

Two local Manitoba events showed that the province was approaching a change, and that influential people were becoming aware of problems in the treatment of mental illness and retardation. The formation of the Public Welfare Commission in 1917 was clear evidence of some enlightened attitudes, and the inclusion on the Commission of Doctor A.T. Mathers was particularly significant, especially since, in 1919, he was appointed Provincial Psychiatrist and was therefore in a position to implement many of the recommended improvements. Further impetus towards the development of a modern mental health system in Manitoba came with the decision to build the Psychopathic Hospital — a decision made before the survey in October 1918.

At least some of the credit for reform in Manitoba was due to the Canadian National Committee for Mental Hygiene and its dynamic Assistant Medical Director, Clarence Hincks. This credit was acknowledged on 14 March 1919, when the Honorable J.W. Armstrong, Provincial Secretary of Manitoba, sent the following telegram to Doctor Hincks:

> You will be pleased to know that the Manitoba Legislature today passed enabling legislation to carry out recommendations embodied in the report of your Committee to the Public Welfare Commission of Manitoba. The Canadian National Committee for Mental Hygiene has rendered our government valuable service, and we wish you and your Committee all success in its splendid national work.

Word soon spread to all parts of Canada of the success of the Manitoba survey by the Canadian National Committee for Mental Hygiene, and over the next 10 years almost every province in Canada would request similar assistance. The findings in these subsequent surveys would in many ways duplicate the Manitoba experience, not necessarily in detail but in their broader implications. The situation was generally unsatisfactory throughout the country.

Again, many shocking conditions were discovered. In the asylum at Saint John, New Brunswick, a certain group of patients on the upper floor were put to bed in coffin-like boxes with hay in the bottom and slats on the top. All boxes except two were locked at night, the two being occupied by patients who had been designated "trustees," with the responsibility of dealing with noisy patients. This they accomplished by urinating through the slats onto the patients' faces.

In Edmonton, Alberta, a novel method of caring for low-grade, mentally defective children was observed. At bedtime, the children were rolled in long strips of cotton with their arms and legs bound, and then piled on a shelf.

In a mental home in Halifax, Nova Scotia, a scantily clad man was found in a small unheated room where he was being kept year round. When questioned, the authorities replied that somehow they knew that the insane man could not feel the cold.

Throughout Nova Scotia a system of county poor-houses for mental patients was found to be particularly unsatisfactory.

> One of these county institutions comes vividly to mind. We entered through the kitchen and I noticed hanging from the ceiling coils of dried apples, which were somewhat difficult to see because they were covered with flies. The Superintendent, who was a farmer, noticed my concern and said, "Don't worry, doctor, we don't eat them, we sell them."
>
> Then he said, "You sent us a questionnaire asking for a list of our patients with a diagnosis of each. My missus and I are short on diagnosis. In fact, we had to look up the

> meaning of the term, and as I understand it, diagnosis means what is wrong with a patient. Well, we did the best we could and here is the list." At the top was the name of a man, with the diagnosis "just an ordinary damn fool," and the next man was diagnosed as a "perfect gentleman." When we saw these men it was evident that the first named was a case of schizophrenia, while the second was an imbecile with a perpetual smile on his face who, like a perfect gentleman, gave Miss Keyes a flower and asked her to marry him. I saw her wavering, so I whisked her away. I didn't want to lose a first-class nurse and social worker.

Throughout the course of his surveys, Clare found at least some good things to counterbalance the bad. One outstanding example was the Maritime Home for Girls in Truro, Nova Scotia, supported by the three provinces of Nova Scotia, New Brunswick, and Prince Edward Island. The girls there had failed to respond to rehabilitation in their home communities, and were considered by some to be hardened cases, their offences consisting of repeated theft, sexual delinquencies, and disorderly conduct. Until just a few years before the survey the girls had been showing little improvement at the home where, in fact, they often learned new delinquencies and, when discharged, were more harmful to society than when first committed.

A new superintendent was appointed to the home in 1917. Miss Josephine Strothard was a deeply but not narrowly religious woman who held the conviction that every girl, no matter what her background or mental condition, could develop into a worthwhile citizen. Combining common sense, ingenuity and imagination in her methods, she, above all, loved the girls and had faith in them. In her first act as superintendent she met with all her charges on the front lawn of the home and asked the girls what they thought of the institution. Not one expressed satisfaction. When Miss Strothard asked about the experience of girls who had returned to the community, she was informed of the Maritime Home's reputation as a school for crime, one where the "graduates" committed the worst crimes and delinquencies.

Miss Strothard then pointed to the flag pole and asked the girls, "Are we worthy of having the Union Jack flying overhead?" They thundered "No!" So one of the girls was asked to lower the flag and Miss Strothard suggested that the flag not be raised until the home held a perfect record in every department for one year. The girls agreed.

The next 12 months saw a level of improvement that was unprecedented in the history of the home. Classes were organized in cooking, dressmaking, gardening, and sports. The girls competed in the county fair in flower display, dressmaking, and other events, winning so many awards for the home that soon they had buttons inscribed "Maritime Home for Girls" which they were able to wear with pride.

By the end of the 12 month period, the group had maintained a perfect record. To celebrate, Miss Strothard invited the Lieutenant-Governors and premiers of the three maritime provinces, as well as leaders in education, business, law, the church, and medicine, all to celebrate in the flag-raising ceremony. When Dr. Hincks visited the home the flag was still flying.

Another inspiring example of fine work in the early stages of Canadian mental hygiene was the contribution of Dr. J.W. MacNeill and Miss Hazel Jacques at the mental hospital in North Battleford, Saskatchewan, where Dr. MacNeill was the first superintendent. The hospital had just been completed when the Canadian National Committee for Mental Hygiene began its survey:

> I was a bit sceptical when Dr. MacNeill was appointed to the post of Superintendent of the new institution because he was a member of the Saskatchewan legislature and had been appointed because of his political affiliation. He had had no training in psychiatry; and I felt that the appointment of a man to the Superintendency of a large hospital merely because he had political influence was a serious mistake on the part of the government. How wrong I was in this instance! Dr. MacNeill developed, in my opinion, into the best Superintendent in Canada. It was my privilege later on to commend him to President W.C. Murray, of the University of Saskatchewan, for an honorary LL.D.

Miss Hazel Jacques was an old friend of Dr. MacNeill. Although young and trained as a dietician, not a nurse, she was appointed Matron and senior to the Superintendent of Nurses, a quite unusual arrangement. Surrounding herself with able assistants, many of whom were patients skilled in various lines of work, she did two things rarely accomplished in mental hospitals.

First, she organized a department of occupational therapy with the aim to involve every patient in the hospital. A huge section of the building's basement was designated for cabinet-making, sewing, weaving, painting, pottery, brass work, bookbinding, and other crafts.

Similar opportunities were then extended to all patients on the wards who, because of age or infirmity, did not have easy access to the basement area.

Miss Jacques's second feat of organization was the hospital's two garden parties and Christmas bazaar, to which all the citizens of North Battleford were invited. The patients sold the innumerable articles they had made and helped to run the events. With the funds received, Miss Jacques bought things for the hospital that the government did not provide: rugs for the entire building, drapes for the windows, pictures for the walls, easy chairs, pianos, flowering plants and even canaries, producing an atmosphere as inviting as that of a country club. Throughout this process, the patients considered themselves her partners and were proud of their accomplishments.

If Hazel Jacques was an outstanding individual, she certainly compared with the superintendent, Dr. MacNeill. Although he began his hospital work without psychiatric experience, he had quickly learned clinical excellence, backed up with a fine psychiatric library. He extended the occupational therapy concept to the hospital golf course, skating rink and bowling alleys, and attempted to make the hospital a centre of social life and recreation for the city of North Battleford.

When asked how he managed to have a golf professional connected with the hospital, he replied, "Well, there is no category for golf pro in government appropriations, so I list him as an Associate of Occupational Therapy."

> I once asked Dr. MacNeill what he considered to be the most effective treatments for cases of mental illness. He immediately answered: "The two W's, work and water." He used water, or hydrotherapy, far more extensively than any psychiatrist in North America and with excellent results. He would leave patients in continuous baths for anywhere from two to twenty-four hours, leaving the patients the opportunity to get out when they wished. Sedation was used very little in those days, but hydrotherapy relaxed the patients just as well. To make this water treatment attractive for male patients, he had the attending nurses clad in abbreviated bathing suits.

The use of work as a type of therapy has been much criticized by some current historians, who claim that the economic benefits to the institution came to be the chief reason for promoting the benefits of labour. This may have been the case in some instances, yet there remains little doubt that the benefits of activity have been observed repeatedly. Hydrotherapy has largely vanished from modern treatment methods, and contemporary attitudes towards the sexist nature of bikinis as uniforms requires no comment. Yet in the 1920s all of these measures were helpful.

Before Dr. C.K. Clarke died in 1924, Hincks accompanied him on a survey of the Rockwood Hospital at Kingston where Clarke had been superintendent for 20 years, from 1885 to 1905. Although the doctor had been away from the hospital for many years, many of his former patients were still there and they gave him an uproarious welcome. He still knew them all by name.

Clarke had been appointed Superintendent of the Rockwood Hospital when he was in his twenties, after his predecessor, Dr. W.C. Metcalfe, had been stabbed and killed by a patient. Instead of placing this patient in restraint, Dr. Clarke left him at liberty within the hospital grounds, hoping he could still be helped or even cured. One day when Clarke was standing on the dock, the same patient threw his arms around the doctor and jumped with him into 20 feet of water. Clarke's arms were pinned to his sides but he was able, eventually, to grasp the patient by the throat and force him to let go. Even after this encounter the doctor would not place his assailant in restraint. Hincks has eulogized his mentor as "the greatest humanitarian in mental hygiene practice that I have ever met. He carried his humanitarianism to such extremes that he was sometimes criticized."

Clarke frequently had patients as guests in his home. On one occasion he invited a patient to dinner along with a dozen members of the faculty of Queen's University. They were not told of the patient's identity. Dinner went off well, and the patient, who was a brilliant physicist, enthralled the guests with his conversation, providing the highlight of the evening. On some pretext, Clarke had the patient leave the room for a brief period and during his absence the professors asked if the guest was to be invited to join the faculty.

> "Not right away. You see, he is a patient here."

The astounded professors remarked that it was a crime to hold such a man in a hospital; they considered him one of the most cultured men and gifted scientists they had ever met. When the patient returned to the room Clarke asked him to tell the professors who he really was.

> "Why," said the patient, "don't they know? I am Atlas, and I balance the world on my shoulders."

Chapter Six

BLOWING UP THE PARLIAMENT BUILDINGS AND OTHER PROGRESS

In April, 1920, Clare became embroiled in a major public controversy. Angered at what he considered to be the unco-operative and unfeeling attitude of the Provincial Secretary of Ontario, the Honorable H.C. Nixon, towards the committee's recommendations to the province, Clare fought back in a vigorous and outspoken manner. After an unsatisfactory discussion with Mr. Nixon on the 7th of April, he addressed the Ontario Educational Association, and his remarks, quoted by the *Toronto Star* for that day, were not conciliatory:

> Ontario is far behind in Mental diagnostics [sic]. The government says "don't knock your own province." Why, we have enough facts to blow up the Parliament Buildings!

Needless to say, such a remark provided an eye-arresting headline. The report continued:

> Are we satisfied to continue with the old assumption that Ontario leads the world in educational matters? Then God help the world!
>
> We're playing with the whole question of the mental defectives in Toronto. We have three special classes for a

> population of over half a million. Vancouver, with half our population, has 16 classes. What I'm complaining of in Ontario is the complacency I find, which is not nearly so noticeable in other parts of the Dominion.

Members of the Provincial Legislature were predictably upset by such outright and provocative statements, and on the following morning, with what the newspapers described as "surprising unanimity," the leaders of the Opposition and the Government joined in denouncing Hincks. The Honorable Mr. Ferguson, Opposition Leader, considered Clare's remarks "reckless, irresponsible and unwarranted." Premier Drury appeared to take the remark about blowing up the Parliament Buildings at face value for he compared Clare to a Bolshevist and Anarchist.

Both leaders used the opportunity to suggest that Clare's motives were suspect. "Men of this character," said Mr. Ferguson, "are in the habit of getting on the stump or soapbox, or any other rostrum they can take advantage of, for the purpose of securing public notoriety and making sensational statements entirely unwarranted in point of fact."

With respect to Mr. Ferguson's remarks, it is interesting to read a letter that appeared in the Toronto *Globe* on the 12th of April. Signed by Lillian Carruthers, a certified examiner of the feebleminded, the letter reads in part:

> If to any one source is to be imputed blame for such utterances (as that made by Dr. Hincks) it is to the Conservative party. The official reports upon the feeble-minded of this Province published broadcast by two successive Conservative Governments sent alarmist reports the length and breadth of Canada. If with the passing years the echoes of these reports have grown multitudinous, Mr. G. Howard Ferguson and his party have only themselves to blame. There was a long period when those two Governments did absolutely nothing for the feeble-minded except to compile reports.

Further support for Clare came in an editorial comment which pointed out that the social problems created by mental defectives in Ontario warranted the use of strong language. The *Toronto Star*, on 13 April 1920, commented that "men and women who accomplish reforms that are worthwhile usually have to make statements that jar the sensibilities of less-informed and careless persons and that seem to slander the community to which they belong."

Clare had good reason to be concerned with the reaction produced by his remarks. The still youthful Canadian National Committee for Mental Hygiene was actively engaged with all the provincial governments in their attempts to improve facilities for the mentally handicapped. He feared that adverse publicity would undermine the governments' confidence in the Committee and hence retard its aims:

> So I called on my friend, Mr. J.E. Atkinson, publisher of the *Toronto Star*. He said, "You are on the front pages of the newspapers, but in my experience the public forgets about news stories in a week or so." I told him that I was not concerned in this instance with the public, but with the governments across Canada .... The adverse publicity might make governments cautious in allowing us to do business with them .... "I am going to ask you if you would be good enough to make an appointment for me to see [Premier] Drury." Thereupon, Mr. Atkinson telephoned Mr. Drury, told him that I was a personal friend and could be trusted, and asked Mr. Drury to give me an appointment. This was arranged, and so I met with Mr. Drury and his Cabinet. I gave this group the entire story of the almost criminal neglect of cases of mental disability in Ontario. Mr. Nixon was asked by Mr. Drury if my points were correct. He replied that they were.
>
> Then Mr. Drury said, "My Government owes you an apology. What further would you like us to do?" I replied that I would like to make a statement for the press of Canada, which would be submitted to him before any publication. This was accepted, my statement was published across Canada, and the confidence of the government was retained.

Clare learned from this unpleasant experience not to make extreme statements in public. Ultimately, he would come to believe that the battles for better mental health were not won on the public platform but, rather, in patient, unheralded day by day endeavours. Nevertheless, another battle was being fought at that time which also captured the public's attention.

For many years reaction had been growing in the medical profession against the large numbers of mentally ill and retarded immigrants arriving in Canada from Europe. In 1905, T.J.W. Burgess, then Superintendent of the Verdun Protestant Hospital in Quebec, said in his presidential address to the American Medico-Psychological Association:

> ... Let me call your attention to another topic ... in the line of prevention of the increase of insanity — the exclusion of defective immigrants. I do so for two reasons. Firstly, because during the past two years the influx of strangers into Canada has been so enormously increased; and secondly, because Canadian immigration laws being much less stringent than those of the United States, our land is being flooded by a class of degenerates, many of whom, if not already insane, soon become so .... Most of our institutions have a larger percentage of foreigners than is found among the native population, and while the greater number of the foreign-born inmates are legitimately there, having broken down mentally after they had earned a residence, there is in every asylum a proportion which should never have been brought to our shores. Some of these have come of their own accord, but it is evident from the statements of the patients themselves that in certain cases parochial boards, benevolent societies, municipalities and even relatives have sent out persons simply as the cheapest way of getting rid of them.

Canada's official immigration policy around the turn of the century seemed to have been based on the principle that numbers, and little else, were important. When the so-called Sifton Policy was inaugurated in the 1890s it had the effect of reducing transportation fares so as to encourage the immigration of farmers to the more remote areas of Canada. Generous amounts of land were granted; it was under this policy that the Doukhobors came to the country in 1899. Canada was urgently soliciting immigrants and free land was its lure.

In his address, Burgess suggested specific measures to remedy the situation, indicating that the problem could be solved by use of strict and thorough medical examination. The Canadian Immigration Act was thus amended several times in the early years of this century; in 1910 a new Act was promulgated, the provisions of which, if strictly enforced, would have assured the standards that Burgess and Hincks believed more desirable.

A startling result of the surveys begun in 1918 by Clarke and Hincks was the finding that the ratio of foreign-born to native Canadians was far higher in the asylums than in the general population. From one particular case study we may understand why this was so. Extracted from "A Study of 5600 Cases Passing Through the Psychiatric Clinic of the Toronto General Hospital," the report reads:

> Maggie C., a woman of forty, came to Canada twenty-five years ago. Her history was that she could not learn anything at school, could not read, and was not able to write her name. Had a pleasing manner though, and like many defectives had some manual dexterity, learning to sew very well.
>
> She began to drink gin and Scotch whiskey at an early age and followed a life of prostitution, finally giving birth to a child. She developed an acute form of dementia praecox, and, as she said, passed through every gaol in London as a result of her many escapades. Eventually was confined in a home for inebriates where she gave little trouble. The "Lady Superior" said that a "colony" was the place for Maggie, as there she would get the benefit of new associations and surroundings, so the poor girl was deliberately shipped to Canada and a place found for her as a domestic. At the end of the month she received her wages which she spent on whiskey and gin, and was at once confined in the gaol, where her mental condition was recognized and she was sent to an asylum where she has remained ever since. In other words, at the end of a month's residence in Canada Maggie became a public charge. Figuring her maintenance at $35 per annum, a modest estimate, she has already cost the Province of Ontario $8750, and if interest were compounded and overhead charges compiled it is readily seen why such people are not a profitable investment.

Dr. Jasper Halpenny published statistics in 1919 indicating that, in Manitoba, both crime and mental illness were more common among natives of certain European countries than among native Canadians. Again, in 1919 and 1920, Professor W.G. Smith of the Department of Psychology, University of Toronto, published a number of articles in the *Canadian Journal of Mental Hygiene*, all of which were concerned with the link between statistics on immigration and mental illness. He reported on one study in 1919 in which 12,000 Toronto public school children were examined; 173 of these children were found to be mentally defective and 60% of these were of non-Canadian birth, a far higher percentage than of the general non-Canadian-born population of Toronto.

Professor Smith summed up the problem and a proposed solution in these words:

> The general impression is that a contribution all too great is made by the foreigner, and that if immigration of foreign-speaking peoples were prohibited entirely, or if they were more rigorously examined at the port of entry a number of these difficulties would be eliminated. The policy of absolute exclusion would no doubt be effective if it could be carried out, but a number of other things would also be eliminated along the lines of industry and production ... the more rigid examination of incoming immigrants becomes, then, not only a necessity but a court of last resort, and the question arises, are our immigrant officials being given time and adequate facilities for the examination of all immigrants and the exclusion of those whose entrance is prohibited by law?

A chief function of the Canadian National Committee for Mental Hygiene was to obtain data and to publicize the results of such studies. Thus, through the early years of the Committee's existence, Dr. Clarke spoke frequently on the necessity of limiting the inflow of immigrants suffering from mental disability. His primary recommendation was for improved examination facilities, both in Canada and at points of embarkation. Clarke's final important address, known as the Maudsley Address, was given in London, England in 1924. Its major theme was the problems created for Canada by an unwise immigration policy.

The Committee published a report in 1922 summarizing its four years' work and its accomplishments in many areas of concern, including immigration. It reported that "the National Committee was an active agency in bringing about the creation of the Federal Department of Health, and has co-operated in establishing a better method for the mental examination of immigrants. Psychiatrists are now employed at ports of entry ...." Although since that time the influx of problem immigrants seems to have been less, it has also become more widely recognized that mental illness among immigrants is not always a product of heredity, but often a result of the difficulty in coping with a new environment.

Clare Hincks's money-raising abilities had become evident when, with the help of Mr. Beers, he had raised funds at tea parties in Toronto, Montreal, and Quebec to launch the Canadian National Committee. Soon after its inception, however, more ambitious plans were projected which necessitated an appeal to the large American charitable foundations where the Committee could obtain more substantial grants — not for the operation of the organization but for training and research programs.

Consequently, Clare visited New York where he met with Edwin Embree, Secretary of the Rockefeller Foundation and later a close friend of Clare's. Mr. Embree was sympathetic to the efforts of the Canadian National Committee, but since the Foundation had never given money for mental hygiene work, he said the request would have to be considered in consultation with his colleagues. Another problem was evident that might lessen the chances of the CNCMH receiving funds in 1920; Mr. Rockefeller had given the Foundation a large sum of money a year earlier in 1919 but, with an inadequate staff, the Foundation was experiencing difficulty in administering its activities. The trustees had therefore decided to distribute the capital in approximately million-dollar grants to medical schools at selected universities, one of which was the University of Toronto. It was proposed that Clare could help his own cause by suggesting to the Foundation some of the conditions which might be written into the Toronto grant.

Hincks and Clarke suggested that the University appoint a full-time Professor of Psychiatry and develop suitable facilities for research and training of medical students in mental hygiene. In fact, they suggested the construction of a Psychiatric Hospital, a project Dr. Clarke had been recommending for many years — but unfortunately would not live to see completed.

The grant was duly offered to the University of Toronto which accepted its terms, some of which may have surprised the less psychiatrically oriented members of the University. The President, Sir Robert Falconer, approached Clarke and Hincks, among others, for advice on the implementation of the requirements to develop psychiatric facilities. The pledge had been worded as follows:

> Resolved that the Rockefeller Foundation pledge itself to appropriate the sum of One Million dollars ($1,000,000) to the University of Toronto for general endowment of the Medical Department upon condition that the University carry out a program of development including the following items to be provided from funds other than those contributed by the Rockefeller Foundation: (1) a new Institute of Anatomy (approximately $500,000); (2) an addition to the Pathological Laboratory (approximately $200,000); (3) a

> new Psychiatric Clinic (approximately $500,000); (4) an annual increase for salaries (approximately $45,000); the program also to include limitation of students to a number which can be adequately educated in the buildings and with the faculty and facilities available ....

Mr. John Ross Robertson, publisher of Toronto's evening *Telegram*, and Sir Edmund Osler, have been described by Clare as "a benevolent Tammany Hall as far as Toronto was concerned." Robertson had played a major role in building the Hospital for Sick Children in Toronto, and Sir Edmund was a Director of the Canadian National Committee. Hincks, undoubtedly with Clarke's backing, approached Robertson for support of the Psychiatric Hospital and came away with a promise of the $400,000 required for its construction; the University would supply the site, and the provincial government would assume operation of the facility. Mayor "Tommy" Church, believed to have relied heavily on Robertson for advice, acted as intermediary in gaining the financial backing of the City of Toronto. The hospital opened in 1926 as the second institution of its kind in Canada, the first being the Winnipeg Psychopathic Hospital.

Clare called on Mr. Embree again in 1924, at a time when the Rockefeller Foundation was ready to consider direct grants to the Canadian National Committee for Mental Hygiene. Before making a final recommendation, however, Mr. Embree indicated a desire to visit Canada and personally evaluate the Committee's work and its need for increased assistance. On the morning of his arrival in Toronto, Embree breakfasted with Clare and Vincent Massey. Massey, who would years later become the first Canadian-born Governor-General of Canada, detailed the history and current activities of the University of Toronto for the visitor, who then accompanied Clare across Canada, visiting premiers, ministers of health, university presidents, mental hospitals, and medical schools. After meticulous scrutiny Embree finally supported the Committee's request for a funding grant, which was duly provided.

As a result of these first Rockefeller Foundation grants — a total of $185,000 over 13 years — training and research programs were subsidized at McGill University, the University of Toronto, Queen's University, and the Universities of Saskatchewan and Alberta.

> At the University of Toronto we concentrated on the Department of Psychology. I felt that the twentieth century would be a century for psychology, revealing to us the

> nature and possibilities of man in regard to his intellectual, emotional and behavioral potentialities. Now [1962] I must admit that my original hopes have been justified only in part. I have seen psychiatry making greater strides. Perhaps one reason has been that psychology has been endeavoring to develop a respectable science based somewhat on criteria of measurement such as we have in physiology ... of course, psychiatry has had a Freud while psychology has not had another William James.
>
> The above paragraph may be too parochial in outlook. It is ridiculous to compare psychology with psychiatry: and I was naive at the beginning of the century to think that psychology would furnish the master key to unlock the intricacies of the nature of man ....
>
> Our investment in the Department of Psychology, University of Toronto, has been worthwhile. It made possible the organization of perhaps the most able staff of any Psychology Department in North America, including men such as E.A. Bott, William Blatz, Sperrin Chant, William Line, David Ketchum and E.D. MacPhee. On two occasions the entire group was offered double salaries to "defect" to the United States. They stayed in Toronto.

The impetus provided by the Rockefeller grants made possible the work of an excellent group at McGill University. In 1924, the Department of Psychology was strengthened when Professor J.W. Bridges and Miss K. Banham (later Mrs. Bridges) joined its staff. The Mental Hygiene Institute of Montreal experienced a similar boost with the addition of Drs. Bert Mitchell and Baruch Silverman. The decision to bring Dr. David Slight from the Maudsley Hospital in London, England, in 1926 to initiate research in psychosomatic medicine at McGill and the Royal Victoria Hospital, was the first official Canadian venture in this field of medicine. (Dr. Slight appears to have been a convincing teacher. It is rumoured that when he developed abdominal pain, surgeons in Montreal hesitated to operate on the chance that his trouble might be psychosomatic.)

Clare's later trips to the United States brought him in contact with Beardsley Ruml, administrator of the Laura Spellman Rockefeller Memorial. A Dartmouth honours graduate in psychology and economics, Ruml was a brilliant man, probably best known today for the Ruml plan for pre-payment of taxes in the United States and Canada.

After speaking with Ruml about the Committee's need for funding, Clare was assured that a grant would be possible. Before proceeding further, however, he was asked to address a group of mothers in Bronxville on the topic of child development. Ruml's wife, who was president of the women's group, would report to her husband on the nature and content of the talk.

> This procedure was now becoming familiar to me. Apparently all major foundations want to "get a line" on those to whom they entrust funds.
>
> At the meeting of the mothers' group in Bronxville ... I related the history of Canada's most distinguished family — the Osler family. I had met three of the male members of the family, Sir Edmund, Sir William and the Honorable Featherstone Osler .... Why were these people among the finest we had in all Canada? The father was a saddleback itinerant clergyman and very intelligent. The mother had a strong character and was the main influence in the lives of her children when they were young. And so I expound to my audience in Bronxville that the early years of life determined to a considerable degree what children would be like when they grew up; also that the mother more than the father exerted the chief influence in early development.

This knowledge had stemmed in part from the findings of a Nova Scotia survey, which showed mentally deficient children did better when cared for by a normally intelligent mother and a deficient father, rather than in a reverse situation where the mother was deficient.

Mrs. Ruml seemed to have provided a favourable report on Clare's speech, for in 1928 the Canadian National Committee received an initial grant of $30,000. Satisfaction in obtaining these funds was no doubt tempered by the knowledge of the work that remained; Clare insisted that whenever foundation grants were received they would be matched dollar for dollar from Canadian sources. Such a formula was meant to ensure the interest and participation of Canadians in their own Committee.

With a decision to use the Committee's latest grant to encourage studies in the field of human development, Clare was inspired to follow the lead of Dr. Arnold Gesell, an American pioneer in the study of child development. He felt that the CNCMH should also launch into work with children. Dr. A.B. Chandler of the Committee staff was capable of initiating studies at McGill; to find an equally competent individual to conduct research in Toronto, Clare consulted with

Professor E.A. Bott of the Department of Psychology at the University of Toronto. There he learned of William Blatz, who was at that time doing postgraduate work in Chicago. To the satisfaction and pride of Hincks and many others in the field, Dr. Blatz would later return to Canada and set up research programs in child development within the Department of Psychology. Those studies would bear significant fruit and make Blatz an authority in the field of child psychology.

William Blatz had worked with Professor Bott in Toronto during World War I. Since the University of Toronto had no department of psychology at that time, Bott and Blatz were working in the Department of Philosophy. After the war Blatz went to Chicago for postgraduate study. It was during Blatz's last year in Chicago, in 1924, that Bott had arranged for him to meet with Clare and members of the Laura Spellman Rockefeller Fund in New York City. By that time Blatz had become convinced of the importance of child psychology and was able to communicate his enthusiasm to members of the Rockefeller funding group, who later provided substantial grants to support the work of Blatz and the CNCMH in Toronto.

Blatz returned to Toronto after a six-month tour of the United States, with the conviction that a laboratory in child psychology was needed. Thus in September, 1925, under the aegis of the CNCMH, a rented house on St. George Street opened as Canada's first nursery school — with eight pupils. The operation of the facility was not completely assumed by the University until about 1950, but, according to Blatz, Clare was the moving spirit behind the formation of the school.

Clare's talent for enlisting the financial co-operation of individuals and foundations to aid the cause of mental hygiene would soon be demonstrated once again. The CNCMH was already receiving assistance from the Rockefeller Foundation and the Laura Spellman Rockefeller Memorial, but it wouldn't be long before a third major philanthropic organization began to play a role in the Committee's success.

> This came about in a strange way. In Windermere, Muskoka Lakes, I had a game of golf with Mr. James Bertram of New York. The next day Mr. Bertram called upon me and asked if I would see his wife at the Windermere House. She was ill and needed a psychiatrist, and he telephoned his New York office that if I ever sought money for our Canadian National Committee for Mental Hygiene, they were to give it to me.

Mr. Bertram had been Andrew Carnegie's confidential secretary for years. Having travelled the world with Carnegie, and being entrusted with the responsibility of giving away the Carnegie millions, it was Bertram who founded libraries throughout the world, and who gave pipe organs to churches on Carnegie's behalf. The large extent of funding available had warranted the establishment of the Carnegie Corporation and several affiliated foundations, with Bertram appointed for life as secretary of the philanthropic institutions. The doors of the Carnegie Corporation were now open to the CNCMH.

It is impossible to consider Clare Hincks without reference to his phenomenal capacity as a money-raiser; he has been categorized as one of the truly great salesmen and promoters of our age. Although it is difficult to put a finger on the precise reasons for his success, a little doggerel written by David Ketchum suggests

> Unlike other prophets who care not for gold,
> Clare Hincks has a greed that is quite uncontrolled.
> Of the pickpockets' college he ought to be Dean,
> But it's all in the interests of Mental Hygiene.

Some indefinable alchemy worked to slake Clare's "greed" when seeking substantial sums for his Committee. He didn't have the advantage of Clifford Beers, for example, who could give potential donors a copy of his book to read — it would be difficult to read *A Mind That Found Itself* without feeling sympathy for the author and an urge to alleviate the conditions that Beers described.

Still, there was no doubting the sympathy that Clare could arouse in an audience. He has been described as the sort of person who can induce a rich man to give a million dollars and then break down and weep because he can't afford another million. Colonel Edmund Bullis, a later associate of Clare's in the United States, has written:

> He managed to get others to feel sorry for him. Tens of thousands of dollars were given him for his projects because the donors felt very sorry for Dr. Hincks. They did not wish to see him fail.

What sort of family life was there for a man who was away as much as Clare? He travelled as much as any of today's executives but without the advantage of jet aircraft. Apparently, while at home — and not depressed — preoccupation with work absorbed him. On Sundays he might take the family for a drive in the country for a picnic lunch, but otherwise, for eleven months of each year, Clare worked.

The melding influence for the Hincks family was the remaining month of the year when Clare joined them for a summer vacation at Muskoka. There he relaxed and came to know his wife and children again. They sailed, swam, fished, and talked; they entertained visitors and relaxed together. Mabel Hincks knew that the pressures would reassert themselves after their return to Toronto, for Clare would again become increasingly preoccupied with his work and she would be left with the major responsibilities of the family.

Clare bought a racing sloop, the *Sewanee,* a graceful boat which was used both for family fun and more serious racing. Bill, Clare's son, recalls his pride and excitement when he was allowed to crew the *Sewanee* on race day. Many psychiatrists and some of the philanthropists of North America would also enjoy sailing in the *Sewanee*. When the wind died there was time to talk. Clare talked well, he listened well, and he told a good story.

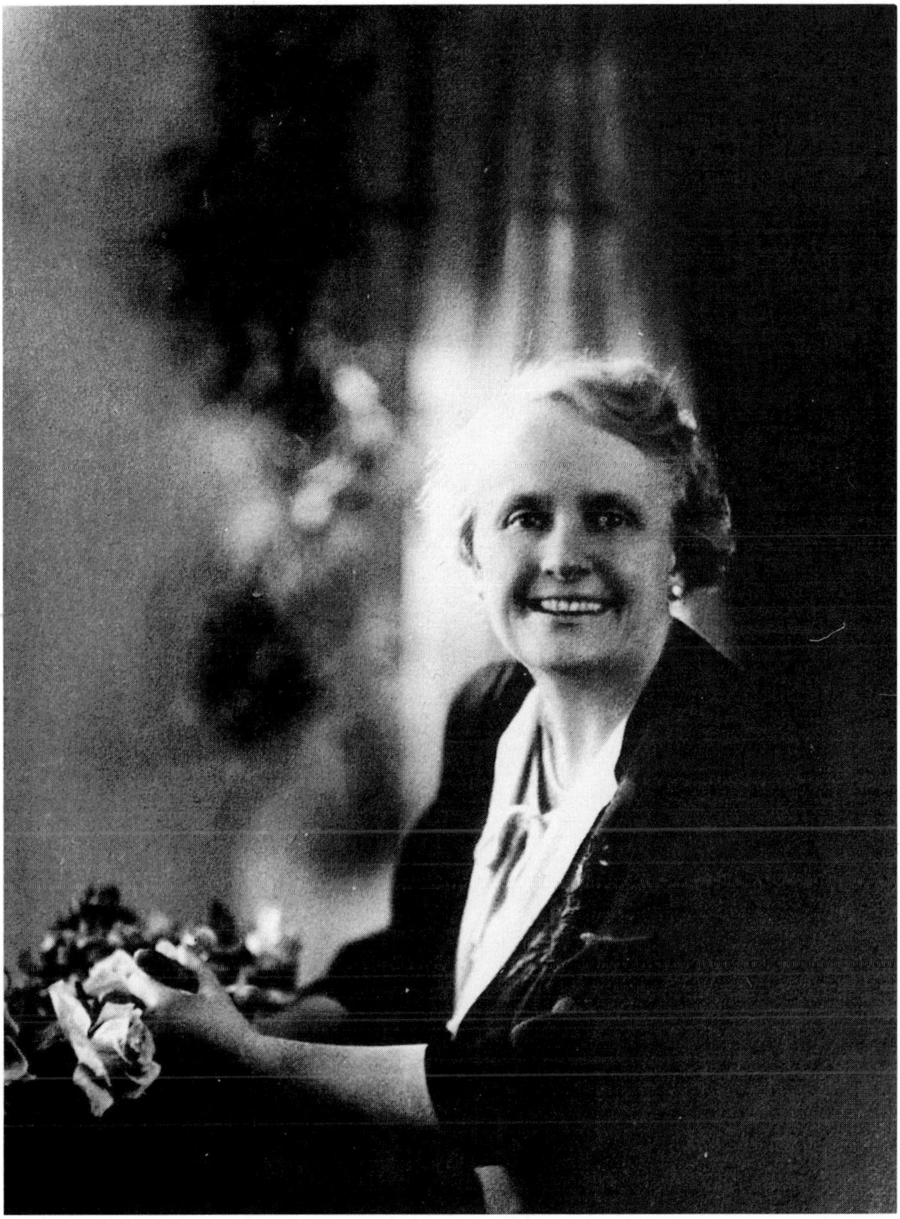

Mabel Millman Hincks, probably late 1940s .

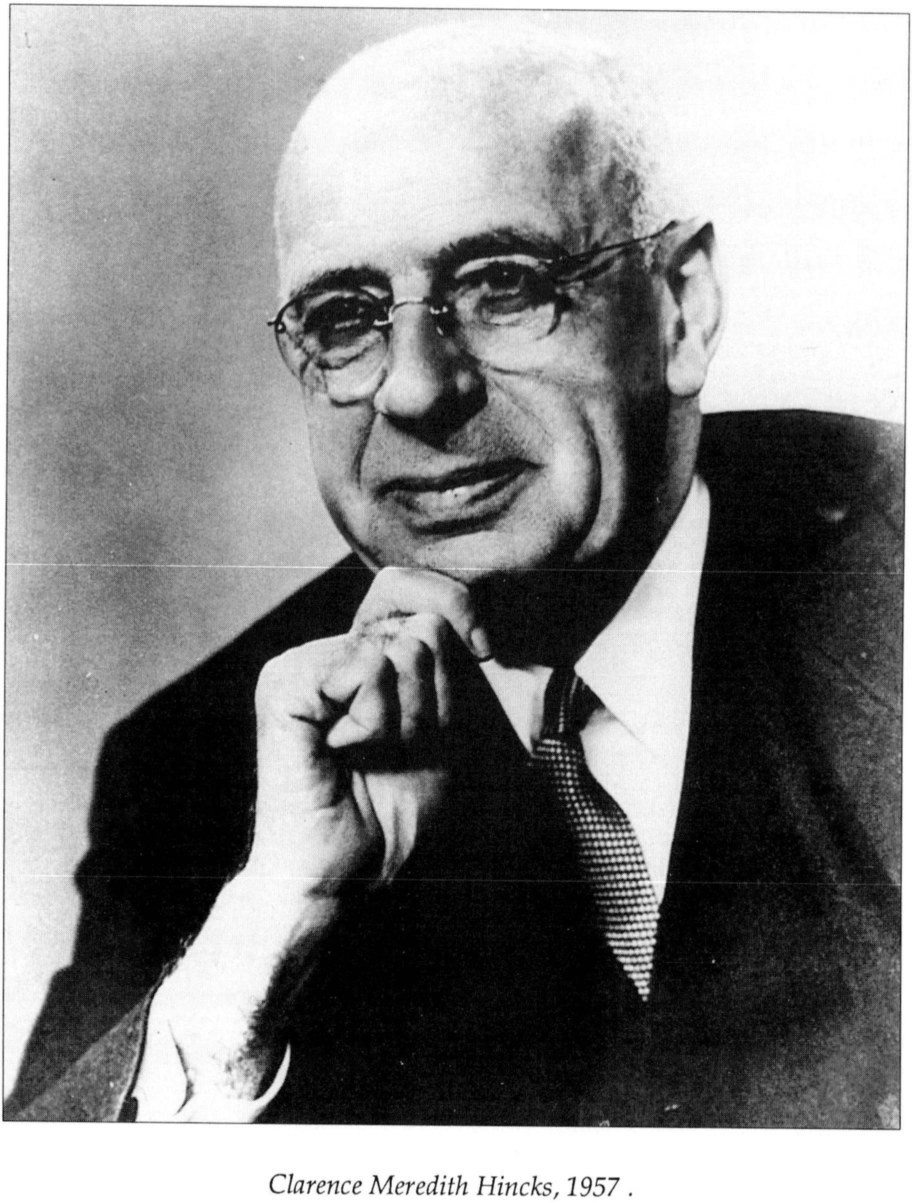

Clarence Meredith Hincks, 1957 .

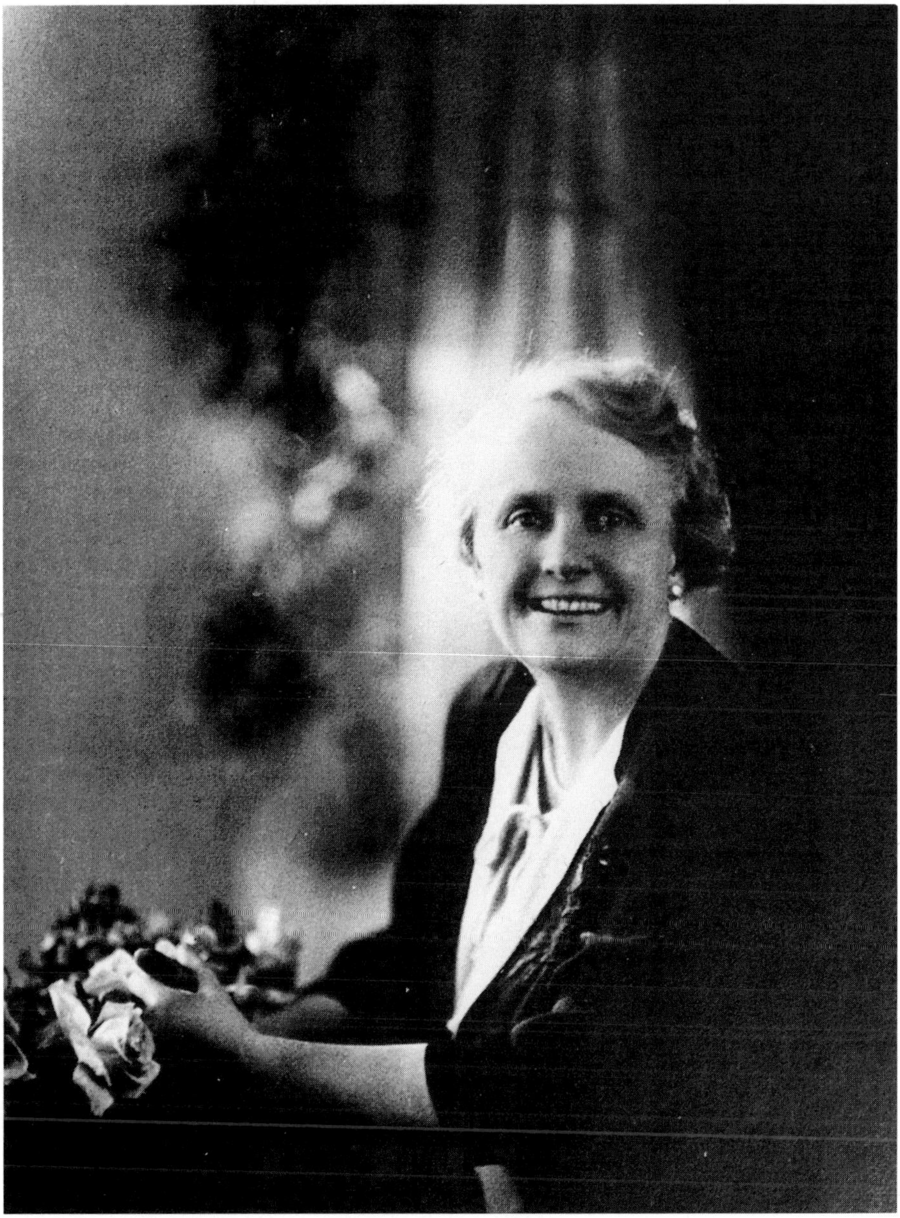

Mabel Millman Hincks, probably late 1940s .

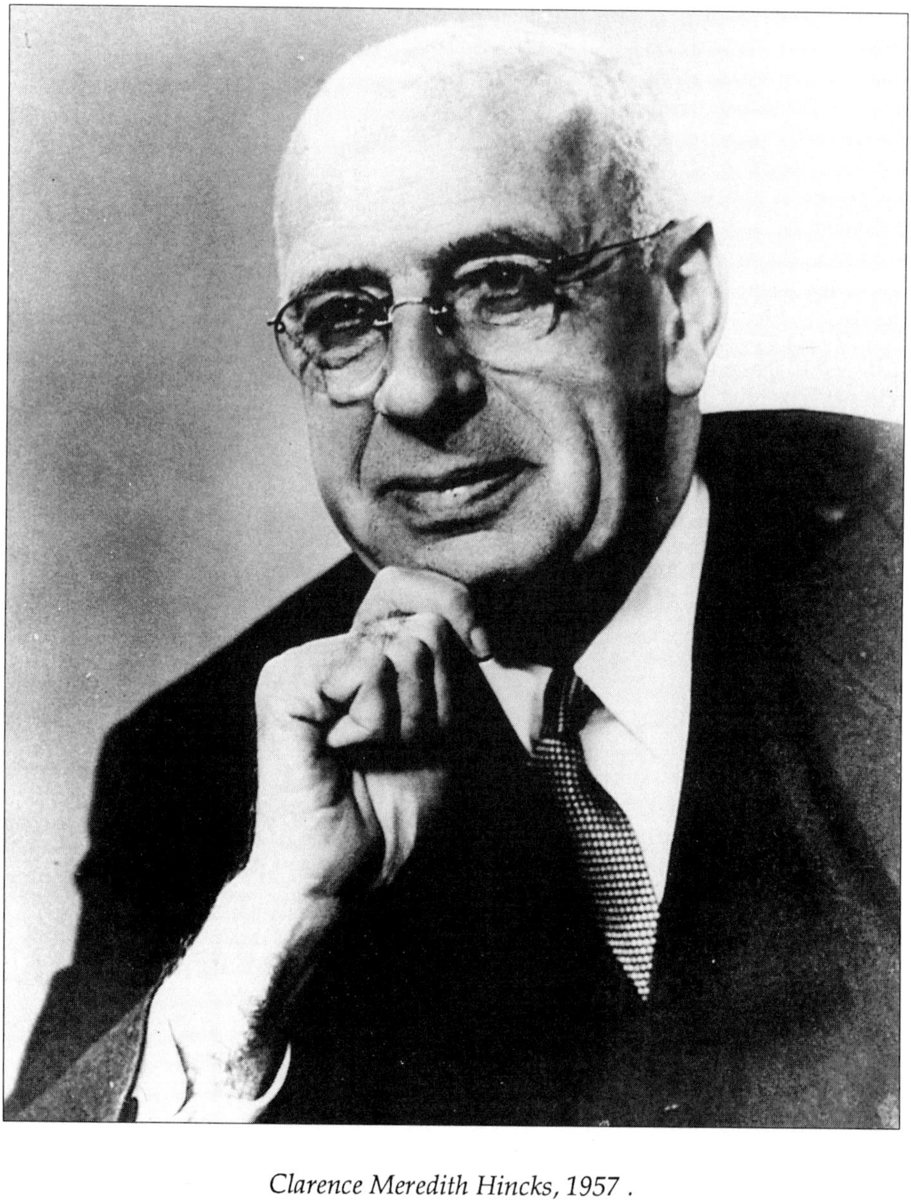

Clarence Meredith Hincks, 1957 .

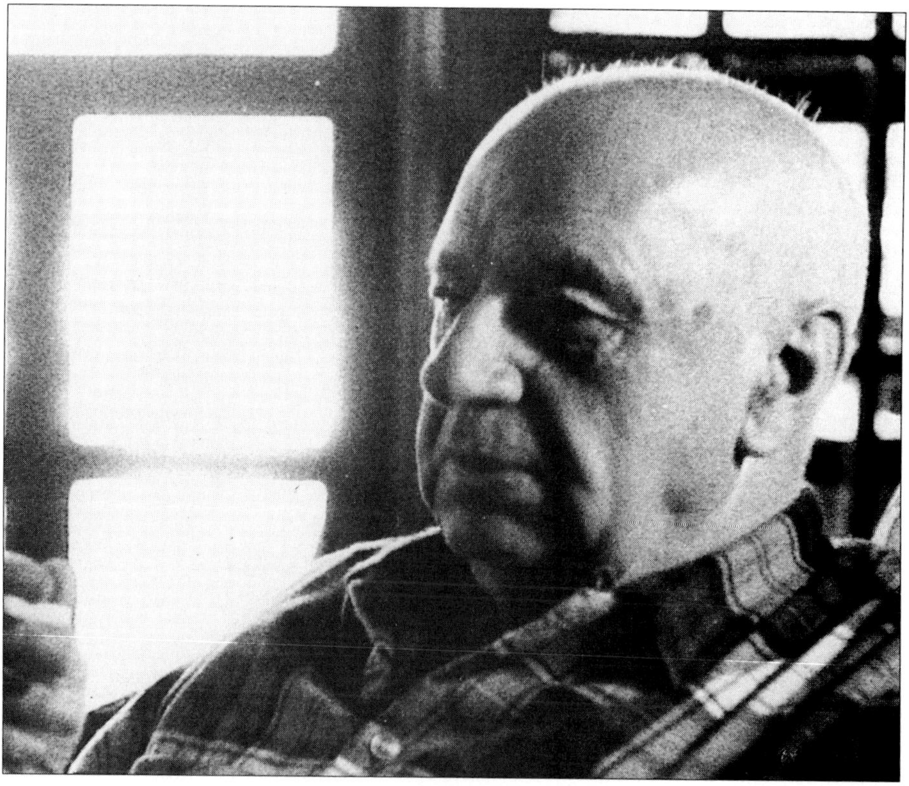

Clarence M. Hincks, Muskoka, summer 1964.

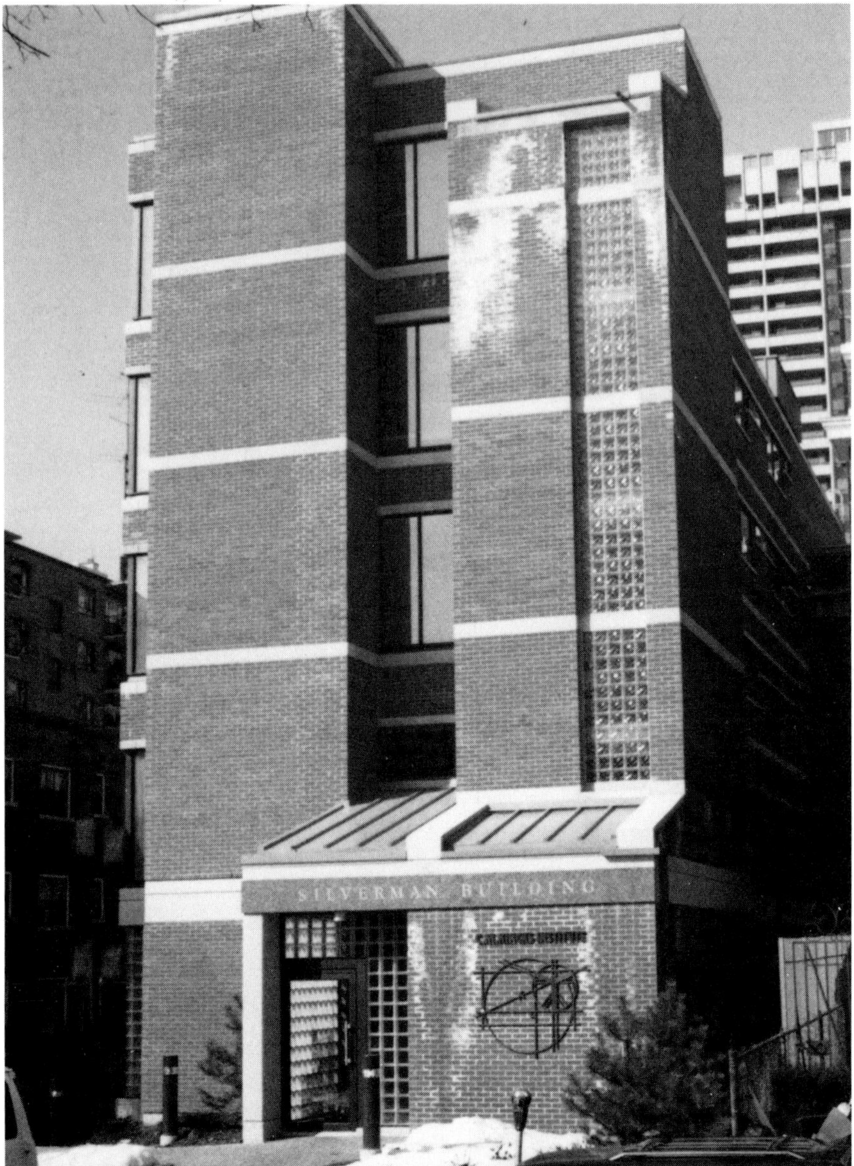

C.M. Hincks Institute, 114 Maitland Street, Toronto

Chapter Seven

NEW DIRECTIONS FOR THE CNCMH

HINCKS HAD BEEN Secretary to the Canadian National Committee for Mental Hygiene from 1919 to 1924, working under the direction of Dr. C.K. Clarke. The second phase of his career in mental hygiene began with his appointment as General Director in 1924, at about the same time as the Committee's staff was expanded to handle the greatly increased work being undertaken as a result of new foundation grants.

Dr. Grant Fleming, a classmate of Clare's in 1907, and head of the Department of Public Health and Preventive Medicine at McGill University, joined CNCMH on a part-time basis, and William Line, Professor of Psychology at the University of Toronto, spent much time with the Committee.

Under Clare's direction, the National Committee turned its attention to mental deficiency in the public schools, the area that had originally attracted Clare to the field of mental hygiene just before the war. With Marjorie Keyes, the new Secretary of the CNCMH, he had time to survey schools in the large towns and cities of Canada, travelling from coast to coast to examine children who were performing poorly in school. Using modified Binet-Simon tests, they identified those children who fell below the level required for successful achievement in the regular classes. Some of those tested had such low intelligence (under 50 IQ) that they were unable to benefit from ordinary school programs at all. Most, however, fell into the group classified as "moron", with an IQ between 50 and 70. Clare and Miss Keyes provided local school boards with lists naming the children in need of special education.

When they began their work, fewer than 100 mentally deficient children in Canada were attending special classes or special schools. Several years later, after teachers had been trained specifically to work with these children, there were 10,000 students who benefited from such classes. As adults, these children became good citizens, often employed by housewives, merchants, and industrialists to perform more or less routine tasks not popular with those of higher intelligence. During the great depression in Canada there was a much lower percentage of unemployment among the graduates of what we now call "opportunity classes" than among the general population, an impressive vindication of the Committee's dedicated work.

Before the CNCMH's emphasis on the value of education for the retarded and defective, such children were major contributors to pauperism and delinquency in communities throughout the country. While the Committee was conducting its survey in Nova Scotia, the government of that province requested an intensive study of 100 families showing a high incidence of mental deficiency. The study led to a discovery referred to earlier, that when a father is deficient and the mother is normal, most of the children will tend to be normal, yet when the mother is mentally deficient and the father is normal, most of the children will show evidence of mental deficiency. Clare believed this was due not only to genetic inheritance but also to the lack of cultural and intellectual stimulation from the retarded mother, who bore the chief responsibility for rearing the children. This conclusion in part persuaded the Alberta government to pass the controversial Eugenical Sterilization Act, permitting the sterilization of certain mentally defective or psychotic persons. In Nova Scotia, some communities had been found to have a 10 percent incidence of mental deficiency.

One of the cities visited during the assessment of schools was Galt, Ontario, the birthplace of Marjorie Keyes. Clare and Miss Keyes called on a few citizens after school hours, in an effort to keep the need for funds before the public eye. Miss Keyes' father, who knew Galt intimately, discouraged them by saying that Galt was a fine city but, being Scottish, was not notably generous aside from the support of its churches. Mr. Keyes was proved wrong; on each of three afternoons, his daughter and Clare raised about $1,000.

Another outcome of the increased work of the Committee in the 1920s was the establishment of classes in human relations. For many years Clare had believed that children are affected by each other more than they are by adults, with the possible exception of mothers and teachers. (In 1938, Sir Frederick Banting held a similar opinion about adult mental patients who, he believed, were helped more by other patients than by doctors.) His belief was strengthened by an experience soon after his marriage to Mabel Millman.

Canon James, who had married the Hinckses in the Church of the Redeemer in Toronto, asked Clare to teach a Sunday School class. When Clare said he had never taught in Sunday School, Canon James persisted and Clare finally said he would do so if he were permitted to have a class composed entirely of delinquent boys. Canon James asked where he might find such boys, and was astounded when Clare told him that he could organize a class from families living within a stone's throw of the church. Permission was granted and a classroom was set aside, carefully isolated from the main body of the Sunday School group.

Clare had remained active in juvenile court work and was able to obtain the names of boys living close to the church. Touring the area in his model T Ford, he had no difficulty collecting eight boys about 20 minutes before Sunday School began. When the boys asked where they were being taken, he told them they were going to a place he had not visited in many years, the Sunday School at the Church of the Redeemer. They protested that they had been thrown out of that Sunday School, but Clare assured them that would not happen again. Reluctantly they accompanied him, and when they got to the classroom one of the boys pulled a white rat from his pocket. They spent the afternoon talking about rats and other pets, and during the next three months they discussed many things, but never the usual Sunday School topics. Clare soon identified the leaders. When he asked them why they were thieves, a leader replied that it was for the adventure. They stole bottles of seltzer from grocery stores, which was easy enough, but it was real adventure, he was told, to return the empties to the store from which they had been stolen, and to collect the 25 cent refund on each bottle. They all agreed. Peer influence certainly appeared to be stronger than parental.

Many years later, a more scientific study of peer influence was conducted by Clare's colleague, Dr. John D. Griffin. He challenged children by constructing in class problems that could arise in the school, in the home, or in the community. In the lively discussion that followed it became obvious that, in pursuit of a solution, the children were affected by the statements and opinions of their classmates. Similar classes were organized in other parts of Canada and the United States. They proved to be an excellent way of teaching the principles of mental health and good citizenship to young people.

Vocational guidance was another area in which the Canadian National Committee for Mental Hygiene was active. Clare and his group had regularly met people who, losing their personal battles in life, had become mentally ill. One of the weaknesses in the mental hygiene program in Canada had been the absence of services to these people.

Later, in 1942, the Canadian National Committee for Mental Hygiene engaged Mr. Morgan Parmenter to establish a vocational guidance centre in the office at 111 St. George Street in Toronto. The demand for service was so great that it soon became obvious it could not operate in such limited quarters. Consequently, the Committee turned the centre over to the Ontario Government, giving Mr. Parmenter the opportunity to work under the Ontario College of Education. Clare did not wish to relinquish all interest in vocational guidance, however, so he arranged with the Toronto YMCA to set up a centre in its main building, appointing Professor Gerald Cosgrave as director and Mr. Frank Lawson as president. The centre has since counselled tens of thousands of boys and men from all parts of Ontario and is now operating in conjunction with the University of Toronto and New York State University.

Another element of expansion in the mental hygiene movement at that time occurred in out-patient clinics. The out-patient psychiatric clinic had been the beginning of Clare's active work in the mental hygiene movement. Today, clinics are found throughout the country, contributing to better citizenship for thousands who need help in everyday living. Two of these clinics deserve special mention.

The Mental Hygiene Institute in Montreal had been founded just before the organization of the Canadian National Committee for Mental Hygiene. As a result of increased grants from the Committee, the Montreal Institute was able to add to its staff Drs. Bert Mitchell and Baruch Silverman. These men, with the assistance of able social workers, effectively served the English-speaking population of Montreal and contributed greatly to medical, nursing, and social-work training at McGill University.

Another outstanding clinic was attached to the Toronto Juvenile Court; it came into being in 1920, soon after the appointment of Judge

Hawley Mott to the bench. Before assuming his duties at the juvenile court, Mott spent two weeks at the Judge Baker Foundation in Boston, one of the leading centres in North America committed to new social and psychological approaches to juvenile delinquency. Upon returning to Toronto Judge Mott told Clare that it would be quite impossible for him to conduct a first-class court without the full-time services of a psychiatrist; he asked him to obtain a suitable man for the job.

Clare's friend and former classmate, Dr. George Anderson, had just written to him from England. Anderson was a Major in the Royal Army Medical Corps, seeking a discharge now that the war had ended. He had just married and wished to return to Canada; he asked for Clare's help in finding a job in mental hygiene. Anderson was ideally suited to meet the requirements of Judge Mott, so after special training at the Baker Foundation he was appointed as psychiatrist with the Toronto Juvenile Court, a position he held until his death in 1948. With the collaboration of Anderson and Dr. William Blatz, the clinic made a unique and valuable contribution to the work of the court and to the welfare services of Toronto.

Perhaps the best example of Clare's good spirits and his undying commitment to the mental hygiene movement comes from a story related by the late William Blatz. On an occasion in the early 1930s an institutional grant was withdrawn unexpectedly, a grant that the CNCMH had been depending on to sustain some of the Toronto research. On the evening following the announcement, Hincks, Blatz, Line, Bott, and others, staged a mock funeral, the intention being to bury the CNCMH. Lugubrious songs were sung, much bad verse orated, and everyone present treated the disappointment with resignation and humour. Clare, who had joined the ceremonies enthusiastically, suddenly became serious and announced that the Committee would not be buried; its work was too important for them to be discouraged by a slight setback. He said he personally would find the money to replace what had been refused them. And, of course, he did.

Clare's first love in mental hygiene work was the public schools, an interest dating back to his time as medical inspector of schools for West Toronto and his introduction to the field of mental hygiene. Although clinical and guidance staff were being trained and mobilized for school work across Canada, Clare felt that in some way teachers themselves should be trained in mental hygiene; the few lectures they received on the subject in teacher training college were not enough.

On a visit to Edmonton, Clare met a teacher who had trained for a year in mental hygiene at the University of Michigan. This teacher felt that the training experience had been extremely beneficial, enabling him to see how his profession could react to the challenge to help children develop, emotionally as well as intellectually; how to help them grow into responsible citizens. In short, he said he was able to approach behaviour problems with far more understanding than he had before.

Clare believed that the Committee should play a more active role in this sort of work. Therefore the CNCMH, in collaboration with the University of Toronto, prepared a one-year mental hygiene course for teachers, and notified school boards across Canada which (at their own expense) sent selected teachers to take the course. The course involved not only lectures and seminars but also practical experience within the Toronto school system.

The success of the project derived mainly from the inspired leadership of Professor William Line, and the vital assistance of Dr. John Griffin, Dr. William Blatz, and many others. Teachers attended from all provinces of Canada and from as far away as Thailand; enrollment in the course was limited to about a dozen in order to provide extensive and individual training to each teacher. The project has been repeated for many years and is now duplicated in British Columbia; graduates of the course are known as liaison officers, to distinguish them from school psychologists and school psychiatrists. The results of the teacher's training program exceeded the Committee's fondest hopes — liaison officers throughout Canada have trained thousands of other teachers. Many of them today hold positions as school principals and board superintendents, with improved opportunities to apply the principles of mental hygiene in their schools.

Chapter Eight

TRIP TO EUROPE 1925-26

Through the generosity of the Rockefeller Foundation, Clare was awarded a six-month travelling fellowship in Europe in 1925, with permission to plan his own schedule and itinerary. He listed a hundred men and almost as many places to visit on a trip that would profoundly influence his career.

Clare asked his father to accompany him to London for the first month. Mrs. Hincks had just died of cancer at the age of 82, and Clare was concerned about his father's ability to get along without the companionship of his wife. The couple had been deeply in love; after his wife's death Reverend Hincks said he prayed to her every night.

Through the early years of his life Clare had been much more dependent on attention from his mother; his father was a busy clergyman occupied with his parishioners and his church. So, at the age of 40, Clare would begin a new and closer relationship with his father. He described the circumstances that brought this about:

> Although I had sailed a boat since I was nine years of age, I was not sure that I would not become seasick on this ocean voyage with my father. I asked my friends about the best preventive for seasickness. They told me that when it first

becomes rough keep a drink ahead of the ship for several hours and then you'll be all right for the rest of the voyage. I had not conveyed this information to my father and thus he was not prepared for my behavior. We sailed through the St. Lawrence River. Then when we got out into the gulf the purser told me we were in for rough weather that night. I asked him if he could arrange a game of bridge for that evening and have plenty of drinks on hand. He said that he would. At dinner I told my father that he would not see me that night, that I was going to play bridge but I said nothing about the drinks. I had a good game and when the ship started to toss I began to drink. At times I could see my father, through a porthole, pacing the deck alone.

The next morning my father appeared at breakfast very white and dejected. He told me that he had not slept all night because he was so worried. I asked him what was on his mind and he said: "I did not know before that you, my son, were a heavy drinker and also that you were a fool. Last night I watched you drinking and saw that one of your opponents at bridge was a card sharp, I could tell by his loud clothes. I am sorry that we are making this trip together."

I then told my father I was drinking to prevent seasickness and that I would not drink again while we were on the trip and also that I would play no more bridge. Then he asked me how much money I lost at the card table and I told him I won twenty-five dollars. When thus informed about my drinking and card playing, my father proved to be a good sport. He said: "Go ahead and drink and play cards as much as you want. I guess my sheltered life as a parson has prevented me from getting to know you and from getting to know much of the world around me. From now on we will be like brothers in confidence on an equal basis." And we were until his death many years later at the age of 85.

In London, the Hinckses visited the Albert Hall where they witnessed a demonstration by Emile Coué. Coué was a French chemist with an established reputation in Europe and America for his success in helping those with uncertain mental health. Using a combination of hypnotism and autosuggestion, he had his patients repeat many times a day: "Every day in every way I am feeling better and better." Before an overflow audience at the Albert Hall, he brought to the platform three of the most pronounced cases of stuttering that Clare had ever seen. He asked each man in turn to come to the rostrum and speak to the audience; their attempts were pathetic and futile. After encouraging them with positive suggestion and light hypnotism, Coué again called them to the rostrum; they spoke eloquently. Clare had witnessed a similar phenomenon in New York City and believed it to be genuine.

In the first of many letters between 7 November 1925 and 29 April 1926 that Clare wrote home, he outlined what he hoped to accomplish while away:

> I plan to divide my time on this side of the water to get a flirting working knowledge of Physiology, Psychology and Anthropology as applied to problems that I want to attack in Canada. It will, of course, be hard to jump from one thing to another. The line of least resistance is to concentrate on one line of attack. If I am to succeed, however, as a correlator in Canada I must at the onset be discursive.
>
> ... I will devote time at the outset to reading, a little thinking and attending interesting scientific lectures.

The same letter made it evident that Clare did not begin with a particularly high opinion of British psychiatry nor of the efforts being made there in the field of mental hygiene.

> I doubt if the psychiatrists will interest me in England. I heard Sir Morris Craig and Dr. W.A. Potts speak at the mental hygiene meeting. If they are representative of British psychiatry, I would rather get instruction from Elton Mayo, Adolph Meyer and others at home. Mental hygiene is attracting lots of attention in England but the bill of fare contains little nourishment. The chief hope lies in the fact that there is lots of popular backing. The chief speaker at the mental hygiene meeting was Lord Birkenhead. It is significant when one of the brainiest men of England will give up an afternoon for mental hygiene. There is need here, however, for someone to direct the mental hygiene movement. They are travelling on a budget of $1,500.00 — Ye Gods! They do not even seem to know how to raise money. Perhaps if they had it they would not know how to spend it. I was not impressed by their outline of a research program if they got a few thousand pounds. They say they want to learn the etiology of mental deficiency — the way they are going about it it seems to me to be a waste of time.

In the weeks that followed, Clare's estimation of England was revised somewhat as he began to see the advantages of studying there. He attended many lectures, and in his letters commented on the speakers and their subject matter. He felt the training he received in physiology was valuable, yet he commented quite critically on his own previously held assumptions of British psychiatry, which were proven false as he listened to the experts speak. He seemed particularly impressed by the anthropology lectures, which, he said, appeared to shed light in many dark corners of his mind. In general Clare was impressed with the high level of culture in England, commenting on it in a letter written on the 13th of November:

> I used to wonder why there were so many more cultured Englishmen than Canadians or Americans. Now I wonder why any Englishman who has not worked too hard, who has had a university training and who is not a moron, escapes being cultured. I have discovered that the atmosphere over here breathes culture. Opportunities abound for self-development. The best of the press is enlightened, good books, good music, art galleries and public lectures are put right under your nose. With a normal intellectual appetite a citizen should become cultured in spite of himself. We have nothing approaching London in America. Boston comes to mind but it is hardly in the running.

Clare was highly impressed by Professor Elliott Smith, a British anthropologist and Egyptologist. He recorded an ecstatic and detailed account of his day with Elliot Smith, touring the buildings and laboratories — funded in part by the Rockefeller Foundation — where Smith taught and conducted research. Clare's acquisitive instincts were, as usual, hard at work. One of his letters told of how he had secured for the McGill school, one of the best nursery-school teachers in England.

Clare's letters from Europe traced his growing scientific and intellectual interest in psychiatry. In a day when there was no Royal College in Canada to set standards or to dictate the time required for study in any particular medical specialty, Clare's training was considered adequate. His self-training over the years, and his experience with Dr. Clarke at the Toronto outpatient clinic were undoubtedly valuable, but Clarke was the only psychiatrist to whom Clare had been exposed for any long period. In England, he was moving not only among psychiatrists and psychologists, but among scientists in all fields; new intellectual areas were opening up before him. In many ways his letters read like those of a university student on first exposure to stimulating scholarly concepts. In a revealing letter written 21 November 1925, Clare commented:

> I have made a pleasing discovery in London. I find that at forty my brain cells are still capable of learning new tricks. As you know, my work in the past, interesting as it was, was organizing rather than scientific. It became necessary, however, for me to turn scientist or to recommend someone else to take over the medical directorship. I do not think that I would have been game for the attempt if it had not been for the encouragement of Mr. [Edwin] Embree and Dr. [Charles F.] Martin. These men said that life was an adventure and that I might as well take on an adventure — into science or anything else. They frankly admitted that I might find myself beyond my depth, however, and if the worse came to the worse I could return to organizing and raising money.
>
> To my surprise I find I like the scientific game better than that of administration. I also find that the last ten years have not been wasted, even in a scientific sense. While I have done little reading and have not been tackling scientific problems, I had been seeing great national problems at close range, I had been developing a great desire to help solve these problems. I am, therefore, approaching my work in London with an avaricious appetite and that is proving an effective stimulus in getting the brain cells to act.
>
> From my very limited study so far, I have come to the conclusion that we are on the brink of great developments in mental hygiene. These developments will probably come about as a result of attacking mental problems from the standpoints — of the bodily workings of people (physiology) — of the reactions of personality (psychology) — and by a consideration of the development of man from the Amoeba up (biology and anthropology). I am learning that we can never understand a mental disease, for example, by a study of mental processes alone but a lot of light is thrown on the picture when we utilize knowledge gained through other sciences already mentioned.

Clare was disappointed, however, by the limited possibilities in England for the expansion of scientific facilities, particularly into areas not yet explored. It appeared to him that the major problem was money. He related a discussion held with a British Government employee who worked in administering university appropriations, in which she said economy was the watchword; there was money to maintain existing university departments but none for expansion. Under such circumstances, Clare thought the mental hygiene movement would have little help for a long time to come. The only support seemed to be from American sources such as the Rockefeller Foundation and the Carnegie Trust, and Clare found that he was repeatedly asked: "Is there any chance of getting Rockefeller money to expand our work?" Nobody had solved the problem of financing such local organizations as the British National Council for Mental Hygiene or the Howard League of Penal Reform. Money-raisers in the North American sense were almost unknown in England; the experience of the Canadian National Committee in obtaining money seemed to astound Britons. Clare recalled a flattering offer from one of Lord Northcliffe's representatives to go to the United Kingdom and attempt to repeat Canadian mental hygiene history. Salesmanship, not developed there, was a Canadian and American art.

Another experience that Clare found both enlightening and amusing was life in an English boarding house:

> It is some experience. My fellow lunatics — I mean boarders — have an average age of eighty-six, four fifths of us are women who are outliving our husbands, some of us I would imagine have had more than one husband. Indeed, to look over the group I feel that the husbands must have had an urge to die young. Now none of us ever talk to anyone else, we preserve the true silent spirit or is it perhaps that we are devotees to that all powerful force of English etiquette? Our only thoughts about each other consists in guessing if our neighbours are as crazy as they look but we have a doctor and he is a good one. His name is Paul — he is the waiter. He is more than a doctor — he is an archbishop who not only feeds our stomachs but gives the whole thing a spiritual meaning. When his patients are on the point of mental disintegration, he comes along with a soothing reviving formula such as, "I would advise a little pheasant Madam" or "You will find the jugged hare very nice, sir," etc.

As time passed in England, Clare indulged in more than his usual degree of introspection. His knowledge, his ability, and certainly his aspirations as Medical Director of the Canadian National Committee increased rapidly. In a letter of 12 December 1925, he assessed the situation and analysed what he thought would improve the function of the CNCMH:

> While my mind is mainly occupied with reading and interviewing scientists, nevertheless, I often think of the Canadian work. With these thoughts my conscience pricks because the National Committee has not as yet struck its real stride. The reason is this — the Medical Director has been falling off in his batting average.
>
> A real Medical Director of such an organization as ours should be continually active in three ways — one, money getting, two, national service and three, research. With my single tracked mind, I was either getting money or planning national service or dreaming about research or worse still allowing myself to become confused by dabbling in the three at once.
>
> When I get back to Canada I am going to ask you all to give a hand in putting our house in order. I would like to be given the opportunity to spend the equivalent of a month or more each year to the securing of money and to do nothing else when financial affairs are afoot. When this work is done, however, I want to be in a position to forget money for the rest of the year.
>
> Our national service at the present time is not what it should be. In fact there has been a marked falling off in efficiency since I became Medical Director. Several years back we were a power for good in the country because we were making provincial surveys and stimulating governments and official bodies to make better provision for the insane and feeble minded. During the last two years, however, we have lost our pep. The reason is not hard to see, we decided to attempt to prevent mental and nervous conditions and this necessitated preliminary research. Our energy was directed almost entirely to the creating of Research Divisions in Montreal and Toronto and making arrangement for Nursery Schools of a laboratory type together with plans for parent education. We had to carve our research program out of our heads as there were few precedents to

> follow. This took time and the national service suffered.
>
> This must be rectified when I return. Among other things we must put a man on the job who will continually travel from Halifax to Vancouver. He should devote his entire attention to keeping in touch with mental hygiene progress and in stimulating progress at every opportunity. This work cannot be done from an office desk in either Toronto or Montreal.

An earlier comparison Clare made of himself to a new student at university, is not entirely far-fetched. Throughout his letters, written over a six-month period in England, he made reference to various new theories, often propounded with great enthusiasm. After later exposure to other ideas, he abandoned his previous thoughts and was off on another trail. Surely nothing could be more typical of the university student as he ponders the rich intellectual diet set before him, wondering which philosophies to follow and which to reject. In one letter Clare suggested to some of his Montreal colleagues a method for evaluating psychological personalities, derived from the writings of Jung. In February he was writing to the same people that he had been all wrong, adding that he had a new idea to replace the old. He had discovered the power of psychoanalysis.

> The last two weeks have been the most interesting in my scientific life. For years I have avoided coming to grips with psychoanalysis. Essentially I am a timid creature, I am lacking in courage. I dislike facing issues and will run around the block any time to avoid an unpleasant task. When, however, I actually enter a contest with myself or anyone else, I am impelled by my unfortunate make-up to fight to a finish. I can well remember avoiding for years the question of religion and immortality. At last I faced these important and vital issues. For two years I devoted every ounce of energy in my being to reading, searching, thinking and experimenting with myself to find a conclusion or at least peace of mind. Finally I arrived at much the same position as Sir William Osler. With him I could say — "On all these questions I have come to the conclusion that I cannot furnish myself with any scientific answer. I prefer, however, to believe in immortality even if I am wrong than not to believe, even if non-belief is right." My two-year fight was worthwhile because I found peace of mind. [5]

Thank heaven my wrestling with psychoanalysis lasted only two weeks and not two years. I made up my mind to accept Freudian conceptions and live absolutely under their influence for the time being. I swallowed without criticism, the view that neuroses were due to mental conflict, that conflict arose because of conscious repression of archaic unconscious ideas, that these unconscious ideas had to do with incest passion for the parent of the opposite sex, that relief came through sublimation. I'll admit that it took some stern self-discipline to accept this formula but Jung made it easier by saying that the incest urge was not really sexual but a desire for spiritual reverence.

Strange as it may seem I absolutely fell under the spell of this school of thought. My experience can be likened to religious conversion. Perhaps it would be nearer the truth to say that I got into a paranoic condition with delusions of grandeur. I felt that I had discovered a key to the human soul, with this key I could unlock the mysteries of the unconscious, the philosophies of the ages and the impelling forces that have created the great religions. I believed that I had a mission in life. I would spend my time in interpreting the Bible to theologians and would start with the Book of Revelations because Revelations is a glorious field for the psychoanalyst with its wealth of symbolism. I would organize classes in literature and take up the very works that in the past had been hardest to explain. If I had time I would also heal the sick and show others the technique.

Elton Mayo had told me before I left Canada how I could get out of such a trance if I ever fell victim. He said, "Read Pierre Janet." I did not want to come down to earth, heaven was too sweet, I did not want to wake up. However, I took a big glass of unprohibited drink in England and read Janet's *Psychological Healing*. I came down to earth and reality with a bang!

I would not spend so much time on my individual experience if it were not for the fact that mental hygiene and psychiatry are going through troublesome times in Europe and America. There is a fight between the psychoanalytic school of thought and those who do not belong to this school. The latter are in the minority so far as thinking psychiatrists are concerned. The leader, Pierre Janet, a man

> who is so great that I want to brush up my French so that at least I can read his work if I cannot talk to him. Pierre Janet did the pioneer work that gave Freud his start. Janet realized the role of psychological analysis and repression in certain cases but his intelligence forbade him making the sweeping generalizations of Freud.
>
> What are we going to do in Canada? If we accept psychoanalysis as it is accepted by its advocates today, we will automatically rule out two thirds of worthwhile psychiatry, psychology and physiology as applied to mental states. Psychoanalysis does not fuse with other forms of thought.
>
> I ask, what are we going to do? I for one would like to throw in my lot with Pierre Janet, and Elton Mayo is his great exponent in America.

A lack of enthusiasm was never one of Clare Hincks's shortcomings; he always had some new scheme in mind to advance the cause of mental hygiene in Canada. It can certainly be said that his continued development in scientific thought remained consistent with his devotion to the development of the mental hygiene movement. A suggestion, proposed in a letter written from England in 1926, concerned the possibility of preventing and, indeed, eradicating juvenile delinquency in one of the worst crime districts in Montreal. He suggested a repetition of the Framingham Experiment; instead of fighting tuberculosis, the movement would fight juvenile delinquency. A district with a known delinquency record would be targeted in an attempt to stamp out criminal behaviour by use of intensive parent and teacher training. A consultation bureau for both psychiatric and vocational guidance would be set up; children's clubs, playgrounds and other activities would be organized; existing social agencies, churches, and service clubs would be enlisted and difficult children would be cared for by big brothers and big sisters trained by the CNCMH. It was a bold proposal but, unfortunately premature. The experiment was finally launched in 1964, almost 40 years after Clare had suggested it.

Throughout his life, Clare tended to be somewhat of a hero worshipper. Evidence of this lay in his devotion to his mother, his affection for and appreciation of Dr. Clarke, and the reliance and affection he developed for Clifford Beers and his work in mental hygiene. In England he developed a keen interest and enthusiasm for the work of Elliot Smith, and later became a great admirer of Dr. T.S. Good, Superintendent of the Oxfordshire Mental Hospital and Director of the Radcliffe Infirmary Outpatient Clinic for Nervous Disorders in Oxford:

> I found Dr. Good one of the most interesting men I have met in England. He describes himself as a psychiatrist, a neurologist and anthropologist. He is all of these and more. From the mental hygiene standpoint his chief claim for distinction is the fact that he has been able with the assistance of his colleagues to reduce the insanity rate of his district. He draws his patients from the County of Oxford and from the city, a combined population of approximately 190,000. In the past ten years the population has been almost stationary. Since the establishment of the mental clinic, the admissions to the mental hospital have decreased. In 1921-1922 for example there were 251 admissions, while in 1923-1924 there were only 207 admissions. I have not the figures for the last year but Dr. Good says that the admission rate has declined still more. These decreases can only be accounted for, according to Dr. Good, by the activity of the clinic. There has been no decrease in the number of mental cases throughout England and Wales during recent years.
>
> It is of interest to note that Dr. Good and his staff utilize psychoanalysis as far as seems practicable with their cases. The fact that an individual is suffering from Dementia Praecox or epilepsy or a pronounced psychosis does not act as a deterrent to an application in some degree of the method. The physicians have apparently satisfied themselves that psychoanalysis can justify itself in a therapeutic way in institution practice but naturally they get greater rewards in the clinic. During the time of visit they were conducting research activities in free association and blood pressure.

One of the highlights of Clare's visit to Germany was his visit with the famous psychiatrist, Emil Kraepelin, not long before Kraepelin's death in 1926. For Clare, the meeting was no ordinary exchange of professional courtesies; it took on an almost mystical aura, like that of a devoted acolyte at the feet of his guru.

> I had two sessions with Kraepelin. At seventy-two he was a vigorous, hard working scientist. As you know before the war he laid the ground work for his research institute and

> had at his disposal several million marks. All of his money has been lost because of post-war inflation. He has succeeded, however, in keeping his workers together.
>
> In the institute Kraepelin is devoting himself to industrial psychology and I found his laboratory a hive of interesting work. Kraepelin told me that he was now more attracted to Psychology than Psychiatry. I think he is changing his work to renew his youth.

Clare's two-day visit with Kraepelin was a high point of his trip to Europe. As a psychiatrist, Clare had read Kraepelin's textbooks in which he had undertaken the monumental task of classifying and describing mental disabilities. Previously, there had been no systematic classification, and most mental disorders were differentiated only by their presenting symptoms, such as depression or mania. It was Kraepelin who first described dementia praecox, later to be called schizophrenia, perhaps the most prevalent diagnosis assigned to patients in mental hospitals for decades.

During discussions on the work of Sigmund Freud, Kraepelin showed no sign of jealousy towards his more famous colleague. He felt that if Freud had been working with the psychoses, as Kraepelin had, instead of with the neuroses, Freud would never have been able to develop his interesting theories. Clare noted that despite the importance and recognition of his work, Kraepelin was plagued by financial difficulties. After his return to North America, he assisted in obtaining a large grant for the Kraepelin Institute.

A final highlight of Clare's trip to Europe was not mentioned in his letters, yet in later writings he frequently referred to the psychiatric treatment carried out by the entire town of Geel, in Belgium. Half of the town's population of 2,400 suffered from mental illness, most having come to Geel from around the world, as their predecessors had been doing for more than 500 years. A shrine which had been constructed in the town was believed to heal mental patients, but over the years it had become apparent that its curative properties worked slowly. Therefore, many who had come for treatment boarded with local peasants, waiting for the cure to take effect.

This phenomenon had been occurring for centuries. The villagers had learned from experience that the best way of dealing with these patients was to treat them as equals. The Belgian Government took a hand by issuing certificates to those residents of Geel who qualified, and it developed a small psychiatric hospital on the outskirts of the town for patients requiring hospitalization for brief periods.

Clare walked down the streets of Geel knowing that almost every person he met was mentally ill, even though there was little to distinguish the ill from the well. While visiting patients in the homes of their hosts, he met a Dutch lady who had been treated in a hospital in Holland. According to her medical history she was manic, restless, and destructive. Having been placed in a single room at the Dutch hospital, she was so resentful at being confined that with her bare hands she removed the bricks from her fireplace and climbed up the chimney to escape. The Dutch authorities were pleased to have her removed from their care when her family took her to Geel. There, with the freedom to take part in running the household of the peasants with whom she boarded, she behaved like a different person. Her case, together with many others that Clare studied, convinced him that mental illness was as much a product of environment as faulty body function. He commented:

> It was only natural when I returned to Canada that our Canadian Committee should urge every Provincial Government to develop boarding out arrangements. We succeeded only in Ontario and Manitoba. Some day the plan will be adopted throughout the country because it is good for patients and it is economical in reducing the need for new mental hospital construction.

Clare returned to Canada in the late spring of 1926, his experiences in Europe having vastly altered many of his views. In one of his letters he had declared that before visiting Europe he had been an inefficient Medical Director and the Canadian National Committee for Mental Hygiene had suffered as a consequence. Although it is impossible to judge the truth of this contention, there is no question that Clare brought new ideas back to Canada; in the ensuing years many of these ideas would bear fruit.

Chapter Nine

DOUBLE DUTY, CANADA AND THE USA

THE SCOPE OF CLARE'S activities broadened in 1930 when he accepted the post of General Director of the United States National Committee for Mental Hygiene. When interviewed for the position he indicated that, unlike his predecessors, Dr. Thomas Salmon and Dr. Frankwood Williams, he believed his responsibilities should include not only planning and execution of the scientific program but also fund-raising, a function assumed exclusively by Clifford Beers up to that point. In a letter dated in May, 1918, from Beers to the chief medical administrator for the Province of Quebec, it is revealed that the idea of Clare working for the American Committee was not a new one.

> In Dr. Hincks, your National Committee has a great asset, one which makes our Committee envious. Though we shall not, of course, attempt to secure Dr. Hincks as a member of our staff, you may quote me by saying that we should be glad to take him on if it could be done in justice to your work.

The period preceding his new appointment in 1930 had been a busy one for Clare. Yet, in the following eight and a half years while he worked in the USA, life became even more hectic. Continuing to hold his position as General Director of the Canadian organization while directing the United States centre, Clare commuted regularly between Toronto and New York.

The decision of the American Committee to hire Clare was influenced by many factors. Fund-raising had become increasingly difficult during the depression years, and Clare's known success in this field certainly played a role, as did his strong rapport with Clifford Beers. Beers had lost his zeal for fund-raising and had also, inexplicably, lost confidence in Dr. Frankwood Williams, Clare's predecessor at the New York centre.

Clare's philosophy on the issue of personal gain in such a field as fund-raising may also have played a role in the decision. He once stated:

> I would like to say something about remuneration to a man, like myself, who secures donations and grants for the work in which he is engaged. In Canada, I adopted the policy of getting my Board of Directors to vote me a salary of one-half the amount I could earn on the open market. I did this to enable me to request without embarrassment large sums from private donors for our national work. I wanted to be in the position of being a financial donor myself, in a sense, and of avoiding any suspicion of looking for money for my own pocket. And I also adopted the policy of never accepting a fee from any patient who sought my professional help. I realized that many mentally ill persons might come to me because they saw my name in magazines or newspapers, and I did not want the medical profession to be able to say that I was using my public position to build up a private practice. Of course, many people would send me personal cheques but they were always returned. I would tell grateful patients that, if they wished they could support our work, but not me ....

One's reaction to this altruistic sentiment must, however, be tempered by the knowledge that in 1919, the first full year of the CNCMH's existence, Clare earned a salary of $4,500. Although minuscule by today's standards, that sum represented a very good income in 1919.

Marjorie Keyes, who would later become the second Mrs. Hincks, had proved almost indispensable as Clare's assistant in the Canadian office. Since she had usually travelled with him as well, acting as secretary, nurse, travel agent, and general organizer, many of Clare's associates predicted that he would be unable to function efficiently in the United States without her. By good fortune, however, Clare found in the New York office Colonel Edmund Bullis, a graduate engineer who had earlier enjoyed a very successful military career. Bullis had just joined the Committee after a period as lecturer on the Chatauqua circuit. Many of his strengths offset Clare's weaknesses; a good organizer and administrator, he was meticulous in regard to details. Bullis would provide the stable element that Hincks required in the American Committee, complementing Miss Keyes in Canada.

Clare promoted many schemes during his stay as General Director of the United States National Committee. Some of these were inspired by the ever-continuing need for funds. With private philanthropy drying up after the stock market crash and resultant depression, Clare focused his attention on foundations that still had reserve funds, and was successful in getting large grants from several of them. Individual donors were not neglected; on several occasions when funds were low, Clare would arrange a luncheon at the Astor Hotel with a Mrs. Henry Ittleson, who could usually be relied upon to donate $5,000 or more.

The first major challenge that confronted Clare in the United States came soon after his appointment as General Director of the National Committee. Barry Smith, Director of the Commonwealth Fund, suggested that they meet. He asked Clare for an opinion on a plan to survey the programs and facilities for psychiatric training and research at all Class A medical schools in the United States and Canada. The Committee's former director, Dr. Frankwood Williams, had not favoured the suggestion because he believed that the medical schools would resent or block such a survey and, because of the depression, would not be in a position to implement any recommendations requiring additional budgeting.

Clare, however, felt that the medical schools would welcome a thorough and competent survey; he further believed that funding problems could be resolved to implement any recommendations the Committee might put forth. He thought that American and Canadian psychiatry was in great need of strengthening and that the ideal place to start was at the medical schools. Since such a survey might take five years to complete and would be an expensive endeavour, Clare said the National Committee could not undertake it without generous assistance from the Commonwealth Fund. In consideration of the difficulty in gaining entry to the 60 Class A schools, Clare asked Smith to host a luncheon for 20 of the leading professors of psychiatry in the country, a Commonwealth Fund event, with Clare as moderator.

All 20 psychiatrists attended the luncheon. They included professors from Johns Hopkins, Harvard, University of Pennsylvania, Yale, Columbia, University of Michigan, University of Chicago, and other schools. As moderator, Clare announced to the group that he would pose a number of questions to each man individually. His first question was: "Do you think that the university departments of psychiatry would welcome a survey?" The unanimous answer was "No." To the second question: "Do you think that surveys of the type we are discussing are necessary?" they all answered "Yes." Clare's third question, "Will you, as head of your department, invite a survey and secure the co-operation of your medical school?" brought another "Yes." Clare then announced: "You, gentlemen, represent twenty of the leading medical schools of the Continent. The remaining forty medical schools will follow your lead. After conferring with our host regarding financing and after we secure qualified personnel for the task, we will commence our job of surveying."

They secured the services of two psychiatrists — Dr. Ralph Noble, an Australian, who was familiar with procedures in psychiatric training and research not only in his own country but in America and Europe, and Dr. Franklin Ebaugh, Professor of Psychiatry at the University of Colorado and former colleague of Dr. Adolf Meyer at Johns Hopkins. The pair surveyed the quality of training and research in psychiatry departments of the universities, together with clinical and laboratory facilities, budgets, and the extent of integration between psychiatry and other university disciplines, particularly internal medicine. Dr. Ebaugh carried the study further, using his membership in a medical fraternity to speak informally with the recipients of psychiatric training, the medical students.

The survey not only furnished a first-hand estimate of the calibre of teaching and research, but also provided a great stimulus for strengthening them. Although conducted during the depression, the study generated large financial appropriations which put psychiatry on a much sounder basis in North American universities. Probably the chief gain was the integration of psychiatry with general medical training, although great resistance had to be overcome in certain branches of medicine, particularly in pediatrics. Several well-known pediatricians published articles and delivered addresses advocating the separation of psychiatry from pediatric teaching. Their position was defeated, however, not so much by the survey as by increased demands from mothers for pediatric services that included attention to mental as well as physical development.

The survey of the 60 Class A medical schools took five years to complete, most of the work being done by Ebaugh. In conjunction with the advance of Freudian concepts, it ushered in modern psychiatry:

> One of its chief results was the establishment of psychiatry as a respectable and helpful partner of medicine and surgery and the other subdivisions of medicine. This was brought about, during the survey, following frequent joint sessions between psychiatrists and representatives of other branches of medicine. And I will always remember with appreciation the participation of Mr. Barry Smith, and the financial assistance of the Commonwealth Fund. It was Mr. Smith's vision that led to the undertaking in the first place. My role was simply that of an operating engineer.

Clare also played a role in developing a system to certify psychiatrists as specialists in their field. He recalled the events as follows:

> When I went to the United States, there was no national system for the certification of psychiatrists. Any graduate of medicine could call himself a psychiatrist and could apply for a psychiatric post in government services. For the protection of the public, we in the National Committee advocated a national system for certification, and one of the members of our staff, Dr. Samuel Hamilton, approached the American Medical Association on the subject. Dr. Hamilton got a favourable response, and there was created the American Board of Psychiatry and Neurology, with successful candidates receiving certification in psychiatry and/or neurology according to qualifications. The American Board demanded four years' postgraduate work in psychiatry at approved training centres, followed by examinations. This plan has worked well over the years and has resulted in the development of psychiatry as a specialty with a status that is comparable to internal medicine and surgery. In Canada, the certifying board is the Royal College of Physicians and Surgeons of Canada.

A beneficial partnership was developed with the Scottish Rite Masons during Clare's tenure in New York. Mr. Melvin M. Johnson, of Boston, had been appointed Sovereign Grand Commander of Masons in the Northern Jurisdiction of the United States. Dissatisfied with the way the masons had been allocating funds to benevolent works, Johnson approached Edwin Embree after learning of his work from a magazine article. Embree suggested he approach the National Committee for Mental Hygiene. There he finally met with Colonel Bullis and Dr. Hincks. The meeting led to further conferences, and in 1934 the masons decided to help finance research into the causes of schizophrenia.

Schizophrenia is a long-term disorder, with little then, or now, known of the cause. Clare feared the masons would have difficulty with the project because hasty progress and encouraging reports were unlikely.

To his surprise, and their credit, the masons were not dissuaded. The advisory board set up to allocate funds functioned for several decades, and although neither the cause nor the cure of schizophrenia has been discovered, over two million dollars has been directed to support research projects of scientific value. The sustained interest and generosity of the masons deserve a fitting memorial.

Clare was an unquestioned success in the USA, playing an important but, typically, often hidden role. His personal estimate of his career there is revealing:

> And so, I went to the United States resolved to be myself. If, according to Edwin Embree, I would fail through such a course, I could always return to Canada. But my plan did not fail. I was accepted on every hand with open arms and made to feel thoroughly at home. I received co-operation wherever I sought it; and I felt that one reason for this was that people felt sorry for me tackling such a big task. If I had thrown my chest out and had been aggressive, I think I would have repelled them. It is true that I made no great name for myself in the United States, but our work prospered; and that was all that mattered.
>
> And so, it was natural that I would develop a deep affection for the United States. I loved it as I loved Canada. I could distinguish no difference, when I crossed the border every week, between Americans and Canadians, except that the Americans seemed to be a bit more cordial. Of course, in the United States, I met many Canadians who had taken up permanent residence there. I found that we in Canada were exporting across the border not only raw materials but Canadian brains as well. And, since Canada is in short supply in regard to leadership, this export is becoming a serious factor in the Dominion. Indeed, I have often speculated about the advantages that might accrue to

> Canada if we had organic union with the United States. Because of the fact that our small Canadian population is spread out for the most part as a narrow ribbon across the northern boundary of the United States all the logic of geography yells out, as it were, for north and south trade, rather than east and west trade. But Canada at the moment is immune to logic of this sort. Because of traditions, vested authority and unquestioned affection for the Mother Country, we want to remain as we are. We may feel in a way that we are "engaged" to the United States, but we are in no hurry for "marriage." Of course, world events may alter our attitude. Economics and defence may be determining factors.
>
> Well, here is my tribute to the United States. It is a country that accepts you, providing you are not a communist or a criminal. It is a country that provides full opportunity for the development of your talents and that pays you well for your services. It is a country that is remarkably free from insularity with few or no preferences for American born citizens over people from other lands, with the notable exception of the presidency. And the United States is so vast, so populous and so wealthy that it can offer wider opportunities for individual advancement than can smaller countries. Despite all this and despite the fact that I met ten times as many people of great ability in my New York office as I met in my Toronto office, nevertheless, I am quite content to spend the rest of my life in Canada. But I will be forever grateful to the United States for the opportunities it gave me to exercise and develop my modest talents and to rub shoulders with its citizens.

Although Clare's memories in later years were fond ones, a degree of bitterness accompanied his resignation from the American National Committee in 1938. Colonel Bullis, who left the Committee at the same time, recalled several factors that combined to bring about Clare's departure. Clifford Beers had become more and more difficult to work with; the days when they addressed each other in their letters as "Hincksie" and "Beersie" were over. Beers' difficult nature proved to be a chronic problem, accentuated by added stress early in 1938 when word came to him that the Rockefeller Foundation was about to stop financial aid to the mental hospital survey program. A crushing blow to one of his pet interests, the news elicited a strong, somewhat psychotic reaction from Beers; he accused Clare and Bullis of conspiring against him.

Clare was also unhappy with the Board of Directors, who had declined offers of research funds because the would-be donors' business interests were in liquor products. Funds were extremely scarce. At one point Beers drafted a proposal to the Board of Directors stating that if additional funds were not pledged immediately, one employee would be released; he, Beers, would accept no salary for the following six months; and both Hincks and Bullis would receive half-pay for the same period. This crisis was averted but the danger remained constant for several years. A final reason for Clare's departure from the American centre must have been the chronic weariness of holding two full-time positions for eight-and-a-half years, commuting incessantly during that period between Toronto and New York.

Chapter Ten

THE SECOND WORLD WAR

EARLY IN THE WAR, medical officers discovered that the number of recruits afflicted with mental disease and deficiency was much larger than had been estimated in peace time. Advice from the Canadian National Committee for Mental Hygiene, and particularly from Clare Hincks, was sought by medical services personnel.

Clare met with the Adjutant General of the Royal Canadian Army Medical Corps, Major-General H.F.G. Letson, in Ottawa. Clare felt that the RCAMC had not learned the lessons of the First World War, especially in regard to psychological and psychiatric disability in soldiers.

Soon after the interview with Major-General Letson, Dr. Brock Chisholm was appointed as the first Director of Personnel Selection for the Department of National Defence. Chisholm later became Director General of Medical Services with the RCAMC, an appointment that pleased Clare, not only because Chisholm was a psychiatrist, a humanitarian and a man of vision, but also because he had served as a combatant officer in the First World War.

When Chisholm visited Toronto, Clare recommended to him two chief aides, Dr. Jack Griffin and Professor William Line, both intimately associated with the CNCMH and both ideal for Chisholm's purposes. Obviously considering the value of their mission to be significant, Chisholm posted them accordingly: Griffin as Lieutenant-Colonel and Consultant Psychiatrist to the RCAMC, and Line as Colonel, eventually becoming Chisholm's replacement as Director of Personnel Selection for the Department of National Defence.

If Clare had entertained any thoughts of slowing down in his fifties, the loss of his two chief deputies effectively removed any such possibility. Far from lessening, his work increased prodigiously during the war years. Recommending his two chief deputies for army service was only the first of many contributions he and the CNCMH made to the war effort.

Many projects were implemented, particularly in the Toronto area. What amounted to a postgraduate course in psychiatry for Canadian medical officers was developed by Dr. Lawrence Kubie, who travelled weekly from New York to offer the classes. Marjorie Keyes assisted in a program to demonstrate the value of social workers in the medical examination of recruits, especially in the securing of family and personal histories. As a result, social workers joined the military establishment. The CNCMH also arranged conferences among high-ranking psychiatric officers affiliated with the armed forces of Britain, the United States, and Canada.

Another significant project was the provision of emergency mental health services in Toronto. Because of enlistment, the civil population was deprived of many vital services; particularly hard hit were the out-patient psychiatric clinics. The situation improved later in the war, around 1943, when the CNCMH secured the part-time services of Drs. Ruth Franks and Daniel Blake. The two psychiatrists held seminars with staff members of social agencies, discussing psychiatric problems encountered in their daily work, and, essentially, training the social-work forces to handle the majority of milder psychiatric cases. While these stop-gap measures were not intended to, and could not replace the work of dozens of trained psychiatrists, their success pointed to a lesson that Clare was quick to absorb: with training, social workers could cope with many of the problems previously handed over to medically qualified mental health specialists. Subsequently the CNCMH stepped up mental health training to teachers, clergy, police, parents, and other groups. Clare was thus able to implement his basic credo: mental health is everybody's business.

In 1941, Clare received a letter from Professor Ned Bott in London, England, on leave of absence from the University of Toronto. Bott described the plight of children who had been bombed out of their homes. A shortage of trained personnel, especially teachers, social workers, and nursery school leaders was evident. Having discussed the situation with Sir Wilson Jamieson, of the British Ministry of Health, it was agreed that anything Clare could do to supplement British personnel with Canadians would be appreciated by the British government:

> I conferred immediately with William Blatz, Head of the Institute for Child Study, University of Toronto; with Stuart Jaffray, Director of the School of Social Work, University of Toronto, and with Doctor Althouse, Director of Education for the Province of Ontario. These men assured me that they could recruit from all parts of Canada a small group of the best elementary teachers, social workers and nursery school leaders that we had in this country. Doctor Blatz and Doctor Jaffray said they would be glad to accompany me to Britain on a preliminary inspection trip to discover the parts of the country that were in the greatest need of help and to assist in formulating with Whitehall a concrete plan.

With his usual flair Clare secured the group's travelling expenses from the Cousins Fund of Detroit and Mr. Stanley MacLeod in Toronto. Passage was booked on the *Emma Alexander*, a ship built in 1913 which, until a short time before their departure, had been mothballed in British Columbia and considered obsolete. Destined for Liverpool, they sailed from Halifax on 21 November 1941 with 43 ships in convoy, at a maximum speed of nine knots. Eleven days out of Halifax, on the 2nd of December, they encountered gale-force winds and the *Emma Alexander* heeled so alarmingly that the passengers thought she would not recover. Several ships in the convoy capsized; Clare had good reason to suspect that the *Emma Alexander* too was unseaworthy. At the end of their painful 17-day voyage the ship was condemned and never sailed again.

Just before the ocean crossing, Clare had suffered one of his attacks of neurosis. As a travelling companion to Blatz and Jaffray, he contributed very little, seldom speaking and never joking. The other two compensated with good humour, however, and provided probably the best therapy that Clare could have had:

> Before leaving Toronto, I had been presented with two matched leather suitcases. Into one, I put a full supply of medication for my neurosis that would last until my return to Canada. This was insurance in case pharmaceuticals

> were in short supply in Britain. For the trip between Liverpool and London, I reluctantly placed my two suitcases in an open baggage car and told Billy Blatz that I was fearful lest my baggage might be stolen. He laughed at my fears and said, "Nothing is ever stolen from railway trains in this country." On arrival in London, however, the suitcase with my medicines was missing and Billy cheered me up with the statement: "You are lucky. You don't need any tablets and capsules. Your neurosis has disappeared." Billy was right.

The group quickly learned the lessons of wartime England: the stunned look of the waiter when Jaffray asked for a boiled egg for breakfast; the sinister excitement of driving through London in a taxicab in total darkness; and the fad of eating raw carrots in an attempt to develop more acute eyesight for the nightly blackouts.

Sir Wilson Jamieson of the Ministry of Health had prepared itineraries for Blatz, Jaffray, and Hincks, assigning each to a different area of Britain. Clare's designated area included Devonshire; there he visited schools, social agencies, and health centres. All three found the same deficiencies and a serious need for trained personnel in a number of categories. They promised to recruit and equip 30 or more women — the best teachers, social workers, and nursery school teachers available in Canada — and to enlist them for the duration of the war. Canada would pay travelling expenses and insurance, and defray living expenses for one month either before or after the work was completed. Whitehall and local authorities would be responsible for remuneration to the Canadian recruits while on the job and for deciding their placement in strategic areas.

Their task in England complete, Jaffray and Hincks sailed for home in mid-February, 1942. Blatz would return later. The return voyage proved to be more dangerous than the journey out; many ships in the convoy were sunk by submarines, seven in one night. They arrived safely in Halifax, however, and quickly set about the task of recruiting well-trained women for duty in Britain, many of whom agreed to work in "The Canadian Children's Service." The only problem was to secure Canadian financing for the project, although with Clare's talents that did not remain a problem for long. Requiring between $50,000 and $60,000, he knew that this sum was not particularly large had the CNCMH been backing the project but, unfortunately, it was not. Unable to consult with the president of the Committee, Sir Edward

Beatty, who had just suffered a stroke, Clare had to rely on his ingenuity and persuasive powers:

> Lady Eaton and a few others contributed generously; and then I had a hunch. Since our work in Britain would help children who had been evacuated from London, and since the Lord Mayor of London was interested, I felt that a cable from him indicating his patronage, to the President of the Queen's Canadian Fund in Canada, would release all the money we needed. The Lord Mayor was delighted to send the desired cable; and Mr. John McConnel telephoned me from Montreal that the Queen's Canadian Fund would give us any money we needed.

With this final obstacle removed, thirty-three Canadian women travelled to Britain and worked effectively through the remainder of the war without a casualty. Margaret Hincks, Clare's eldest daughter, was one of the volunteers. Whitehall and local British authorities were thoroughly pleased with their activities. With William Blatz's help, the children's services contingent established a nursery school system throughout the country, a system that remains in effect to this day.

Chapter Eleven

THE POST-WAR YEARS

THE POST-WAR YEARS were punctuated by a number of events in the mental hygiene field: a great expansion of the work of the Canadian National Committee across Canada; the development of the World Federation for Mental Health; the change of name from the CNCMH to the Canadian Mental Health Association in 1950; close co-operation with the Canadian Broadcasting Corporation; establishment of a nationwide Mental Health Week; consultation with the National Film Board in the production of mental health films; increased attention to the mental health needs of older citizens; participation in the development of the Canadian Psychiatric Association; a mental health survey of Newfoundland, in 1949; and the promotion of research.

By the end of the war Clare was 62 years old. Although to a man of his accustomed vigour and vitality this was not particularly old, he realized he was no longer young and flexible enough to change his ways. Since 1918, he had been functioning essentially as a free agent, particularly during the years following C.K. Clarke's death in 1924 when Clare assumed directorship of the Canadian National Committee. Primarily a field man, he had often lived out of a suitcase for long periods at a time, yet over the years he was fortunate to have had the co-operation and assistance of a number of particularly able individuals. They included Dr. Jack Griffin (his successor as General Director of the Canadian Mental Health Association), Professor William Line, Dr. Grant Fleming, Mr. Jack Seeley, Mr. D.M. LeBourdais, and Dr. Harry Spaulding. Although constitutionally responsible to the President of the Committee, Sir Edward Beatty, Clare had been free to develop programs without the necessity of clearance through committees and sub-committees. He freely sought the partnership and confidence of all levels of government, and he usually got what he wanted, believing he received this co-operation because governments knew he could be trusted not to reveal their administrative weaknesses to the press or to the public at large.

> I knew that governments were afraid of me because of the possibility that I might take the public into my confidence and, no doubt, this fear was a factor in governments' complying with our recommendations. With the confidence of governments, we were called upon to recruit leaders for strategic governmental health posts. One reason I never exposed governmental weaknesses in our field was because I did not want to frighten patients away from mental hospital treatment even although our hospitals were not ideal.

Another of his policies was to maintain the anonymity of himself and the organization as much as possible. He sought improvements in mental health, not the aggrandizement of the Canadian Mental Health Association. When any improvement was accomplished he gave full credit to the government, the university, or whatever organization had been responsible — never to the CMHA. This, he believed, was not altruism but simply good business.

The pattern of planning followed by Clare and his colleagues before the war had led to many achievements in the mental health field. Included among these advances were the following:

- the improvement of public attitudes towards patients in mental institutions
- emphasis on treatment rather than custody as the chief aim of mental institutions
- introduction into Canada of the Binet-Simon intelligence tests
- inauguration of the first mental health clinic in a Canadian general hospital

- psychiatric screening of immigrants under the auspices of the federal government
- compilation of annual statistics relating to mental hospitals
- development of the first university institute for child study, with the assistance of Dr. William Blatz; initiation in Canada of parent education on child development; the creation of nursery schools
- participation in the founding of the Toronto Psychiatric Hospital and the development of the Allen Memorial Institute in Montreal; detection of mentally deficient children in Canadian public schools; persuasion of school boards to provide special classes and special schools for these children
- provision of the first one-year training course in mental health in Canada for a group of selected school teachers from across the country
- employment in Canada of the first full-time specialist in psychosomatic medicine in a general teaching hospital
- development of the first vocational guidance centre in Canada
- study of all mental hospitals in Canada, a program which led to substantial improvements in organization and patient care
- acquisition of government support in several Canadian provinces for boarding-out care of discharged mental hospital patients
- employment of social workers in mental hospitals
- provision of financial support to professors in several Canadian universities for research and teaching in mental health.

When Clare reviewed this partial list of Committee achievements, he considered the venture to have been a successful one. Given the Committee's previous success, he felt that future work should continue as it had in the past, without any profound change in direction. He compared his position at that point in his career with that of his former neighbour in St. Marys and founder of the famous Canadian department store, Timothy Eaton. Retired from active leadership of the enterprise, Eaton had given his son, Jack, control of the business at a time when the company consisted of a large Toronto retail store and a major mail order business. Soon after succeeding his father, Jack began expansion, obtaining land in Winnipeg for another retail store. Clare and the senior Mr. Eaton often spoke about the difficulty of retirement for men who had been in control during their active careers. Eaton was disturbed to see his successful business being changed, and Clare realized he felt the same way about the CNCMH. He, similarly, advocated caution when his successor, Jack Griffin, supported a tremendous expansion of the Committee's work:

> Jack was right but I was not 100 percent wrong in dragging my feet. You see, Jack had a vision of seeing our organization with divisions in every province, with hundreds of local branches, with tens of thousands of members and with the battle cry: "Mental Health is Everybody's Business." To a considerable extent, Jack brought about this miracle, with one province rivaling the Red Cross in strength, program, and support.
>
> Now, why did I drag my feet? Well, I had the conviction that reforms and progress in our field depended upon continuous surveys; and upon the integration of our work with social work, medical, educational, clinical, legal and industrial forces, with these forces and governments getting all the credit for progress while our national organization would be known merely as a catalyzer and stimulator. I was afraid that, by developing a large mental health organization, we would be focusing our attention on our expansion and not primarily on the mental health programs that beset us at every side. And I wondered where we would get the informed, dynamic leadership that would be necessary for a multiplicity of divisions and branches. Without sound and expert leadership a huge organization could not function adequately.

Before long, however, Clare agreed to Griffin's plans. In February, 1950, the CNCMH passed a by-law changing its name to the Canadian Mental Health Association and then chose a distinctive symbol to represent the organization — a white cross set on a blue background.

One of the association's first major moves under its new policy was the formation of a provincial division in Ontario, a project funded by the Atkinson Charitable Foundation. Mr. J.D. Parks, the newly appointed Executive Director of the first provincial association, gained the assistance of the Women's Institute of Ontario and the active participation of its many branch members. At rural branch meetings of the Institute, speakers expanded upon the mental health issues addressed by the association, and volunteers distributed literature to the public. The local women's groups helped Mrs. Kathleen Hilliker of the Ontario division's staff to develop what was called "Penny Roundup," a new idea for fund-raising which had come from a staff member of Toronto's Ryerson Institute, Mr. Parker, who had observed that people too busy to take their loose pennies to the bank instead often allowed them to accumulate in jars and boxes at home. J.D. Parks and Mrs. Hilliker arranged for mental hospital patients to produce Penny Roundup bags, which, along with mental health pamphlets, were distributed through branches of the Women's Institute and other organizations throughout the province. Thousands of dollars of new income were harvested for promotion of the mental health cause, and many new and permanent supporters were enlisted for the Canadian Mental Health Association, making it possible to mount an increasingly effective program of public education.

The White Cross Open Door Service was reminiscent of one of Clare's early psychiatric outpatient clinics which had operated just before and after the First World War. Designed to offer assistance to those experiencing personal or family mental health problems, the open-door service provided initial consultation and, when necessary, referral to suitable sources of professional help. It did not offer long-term treatment programs; these services were available at other clinics and hospitals and from private physicians. Yet, without any advertising, the Open Door Service attracted more clients than it could effectively handle, including many from outside Toronto. People sought help for the same types of problems they would bring to any mental health clinic — marital difficulties, delinquencies and early mental illness. With Marjorie Keyes as principal worker, the Open Door Service fulfilled a previously unmet need. It was the success of the White Cross enterprise that convinced Clare of the need for Association branches across Canada.

Another study during these post-war years investigated the mental health of senior citizens. In 1952, Mr. James Pryce and Mr. C.S. Lusk of the T. Eaton Company called on Clare at the CMHA office in Toronto. The company was facing a problem with many of its retiring employees, who, as they approached the end of their employment years, became increasingly disturbed. Although a reduction in income was a reality of retirement, poverty was not the difficulty these people faced; their lives felt empty of emotional and spiritual enjoyment. Clare brought the issue to the Association which, in collaboration with the company, designed a program to suit the needs of those employees approaching retirement. Entitled "Preparing for the Next Ten Years," the program consisted of a dozen afternoon meetings each year devoted to topics like health, recreation, hobbies, economics, and human adjustment. Open to employees and former employees, the meetings were enlivened by free discussion, with retired men and women sharing details of their lives after employment.

Clare also played a role in the development of the World Federation for Mental Health. This was a logical sequel to his association with Clifford Beers in 1930 when the International Committee for Mental Hygiene was organized, Clare having also participated in the first International Congress on Mental Hygiene held in Washington in the same year. Following World War II, the World Federation for Mental Health replaced the pioneering International Committee, and in 1954 Canada hosted the Fifth International Congress in Toronto, when more than 2,000 delegates from 55 countries attended. Clare credited much of the success of this event to his colleague, Professor William Line, a past-president of the World Federation, who was responsible for program planning:

> To me, it was a thrill to rub shoulders with men and women from all over the world who were working to promote mental health; and I was particularly interested in the delegation from Soviet Russia. I had said at the first International Congress held in Washington that mental health forces should combat war, and when I conferred with Soviet delegates in Toronto, I felt that with a world-wide movement we could certainly contribute to the establishment of permanent peace.

Before the war the use of mass communication by the National Committee was limited. After 1943, however, the association received as much publicity as it required — on radio, in documentary film and later in television. Media producers had discovered the appeal of the CMHA story, and the public was eager for information on human development, mental disabilities, delinquency, and mental health needs. The Canadian Broadcasting Corporation, in partnership with the CMHA, produced "Radio School for Parents," three series of dramas entitled "In Search of Ourselves," and the series "Life with the Robinsons." Jack Griffin produced a film on "Classes in Human Relations in an Elementary School Setting." Radio, television, film, and the press had become allies of the CMHA.

Chapter Twelve

CLARE HINCKS AND HIS FAMILY

THROUGHOUT THIS ACCOUNT of Clare's story, his personal life scarcely emerges. Three children were born during his first marriage. He married again after the death of his first wife and eventually grandchildren appeared. Yet I have left these incidents for a final chapter precisely because they were, for Clarence Hincks, almost mere incidents; his wife and family did not reside in the centre of his life. For most of the year mental hygiene was his central concern, his family, peripheral.

Clare's first wife, Mabel Millman, was born on 30 October 1885, in Kingston, Ontario. Her father, Thomas Millman, was Assistant Medical Superintendent at Rockwood Asylum, where C.K. Clarke was superintendent. Mabel was the second of five children, four of whom were girls. The Millmans moved to Toronto in 1888.

Mabel had always been an exceptional student and graduated with the gold medal from Havergal College. After a year of study in Switzerland she enrolled at the University of Toronto, where she was again a gold medallist on receipt of her BA in 1907. She then won a scholarship to study for a year at Bryn Mawr College near Philadelphia.

During the interval between college life and marriage, Mabel worked as a translator for an insurance company (she had studied languages). She taught part-time and assisted a University of Toronto professor correcting essays. On 12 September 1912 she married Clare Hincks; of their courtship we have no information.

In the early years of her marriage Mrs. Hincks, of necessity, supplemented the family income. On 3 November 1916 she gave birth to Margaret Maude, the first of three Hincks children. Norman William arrived on 4 February 1919 — Clare was away at the time — and Barbara Mary on 26 December 1927.

All three of Hincks's children remember his enthusiasm with his work, though this also meant they rarely saw him. During the 1930s, when he worked in both Canada and the USA, he often would only appear at home to take the family for picnic outings on Sunday afternoons. Although Barbara, the youngest of the family, has suggested that her father was never at ease with small children, she also recalls her enjoyment of the Sunday outings.

The annual month-long family vacation, usually taken in August, left a favourable impression with the children. At Muskoka their father's gift as a raconteur, host, dining-room clown, and sailing expert could all be displayed to their fullest without the distraction of his work. His vivid descriptions of places he had visited and people he knew, given with a touch of exaggeration or caricature, made good stories. When the children had retired for the evening he entertained the adults with further tales, earthy yet never salacious.

Visitors often shared the family cottage on Lake Rosseau. Friends and colleagues of Clare's came from other parts of Canada and the United States, sometimes staying at "Nibwakawin," a large house owned by Marjorie Keyes and operated on a semi-commercial basis as a summer hostel for visitors in the mental hygiene or related fields. When business concerns entered the cottage conversation, discussion was easy-going, the hard work and unrelenting task of raising money usually forgotten. A specialty of Clare's while at Muskoka was the "Lake Rosseau Cocktail." In the middle of a pleasant outing on the lake, Clare would suddenly stop the motor or furl the sail and with a mysterious air he would delve into a hidden locker, finally to emerge with a flourish, producing a battered cup and a bottle of rye. A generous scoop of water was then transformed into a Lake Rosseau cocktail, shared by all in the boat from a common cup.

All Clare's children recall his fascinating conversational ability. Quite unintentionally and without any evidence of egotism, Clare apparently dominated talk at the dinner table. Although much of it concerned psychology and psychiatry, which might seem to have been beyond the comprehension of youngsters, Margaret recalls that she obtained a scholarship in psychology at the University of Toronto almost without effort, because the concepts were completely familiar to her and were part of her thinking before she ever reached university.

Clare's influence on his family did not always lead to a successful academic future for his children, however. Both Margaret and Bill began to study medicine at the University of Toronto inspired by their father's ideals, yet neither completed the course. Margaret became a teacher in the Toronto school system; Bill spent many years in the ministry of the United Church as a missionary in Africa; Barbara became a housewife and mother.

It is impossible to assess Clare's marriage to Mabel Millman. We know that she raised the children almost unaided, and her social life was limited largely to Clare's friends and professional acquaintances. In accordance with social convention it was nearly impossible to invite friends to the house for an evening, since Clare was away so much of the time. To compensate for the isolation she immersed herself in community activities, playing an active role in the religious education of children. Mabel served in the 1920s as president of the Toronto School of Religious Education for Children's Workers, and in the 1930s as president of the Toronto Religious Education Council. For over 30 years she served on the board of the Children's Aid Society.

Clare's illness created added stress for his family. His children never understood his episodes of depression, and it is doubtful that Mabel Hincks did either. With each episode of depression, heralded by a period of withdrawal, he would remain silent and moody at home, or would disappear to a third floor room at the College Street offices until the illness subsided. Even in the relaxed atmosphere of Muskoka he preferred to sleep and work in a small room above the boathouse.

In the 1940s, Mabel Hincks began to suffer increasingly with arthritis in her legs. In the early part of 1951, severe pain finally induced her physicians to perform a sympathectomy, severing some of the nerve supply to the legs. Post-operative pneumonia complicated her convalescence, and a fatal reaction to a drug brought her death on 17 March 1951. She and Clare had been married for 38 years and were both 65 years old at the time of her death.

In 1952, the year following Mabel's death, Clare handed the general directorship of the Canadian Mental Health Association to Jack Griffin. He did not retire, however; he remained as a consultant and continued full-time activities, giving up only some of the worries and responsibilities that had consumed so much of his time.

In 1957 Clare approached each of his children with an unusual request; he wished to remarry, but sought their approval first. Many years later he laughed heartily as he wondered what he would have done if they had answered no; none did, and he married Marjorie Keyes.

Marjorie Keyes had been born in Toronto in 1893. After completing high school and deciding to become a nurse, she trained at the Toronto General Hospital and graduated in 1915. During the final segment of her training she began work with the Social Service Department of the Toronto General Hospital and the Psychiatric Out-Patient Clinic run by C.K. Clarke and his assistants Clare Hincks and O.C.J. Withrow. Miss E. De V. Clarke, the clinic's nurse and psychiatric social worker, left soon after the war began to join the nursing staff of No. 4 Canadian General Hospital, organized by her father to serve in France.

After graduation Miss Keyes joined the clinic full-time, replacing Miss Clarke. Several years later, a generous gift from Mrs. D.A. Dunlap enabled her to spend four months studying in the USA, and although she rejoined the clinic on her return from the United States, she was soon asked to join the newly founded CNCMH. There, she and Clare remained as the only full-time staff for some time.

Marjorie Keyes participated in the first hospital survey in Manitoba, and for the next 40 years would prove to be an extremely valuable member of the Committee team. Vitally important to Clare, she protected him during his depressed episodes, transcribed his letters and speeches, organized his appointments, acted as hostess for visitors to the CNCMH offices, assisted in the major surveys, and, during Clare's tenure as head of the American committee, acted as his liaison with the staff and the Committee's work in Canada.

Clare's and Marjorie Keyes' relationship was obviously close. Consequently, it could not have come as a great surprise to family and friends when, in 1957, six years after Mabel Hincks's death, Marjorie Keyes became the second Mrs. Hincks.

Clare's activities in mental hygiene subsided after 1957. He remained as official Consultant to the CMHA, but did little active work, particularly in the 1960s. Towards the close of his life, however, Clare was honoured for his many years of dedication to the mental health movement. In 1953, he received the Coronation Medal; in 1954, the Mental Health Award from the Montreal Mental Hygiene Institute, and in 1957, a D.Sc. (*Honoris causa*) from the University of British Columbia. In what must have been in his own mind the culmination of his career, Clare received an honorary LLD from his *alma mater*, the University of Toronto, in November 1963.

It was on the occasion of a dinner to commemorate this award that I first met Clare Hincks. He was in good form that night. With many of his old friends in attendance, good cheer permeated the atmosphere. Clare was vibrant, responding to toasts with ease and humour, aglow with energy and camaraderie. He was then 78 but carried his years without effort. Some months later we met again for a lengthy conversation, an encounter which lacked the stimulus that had stirred him to his earlier heights. He seemed older but, nonetheless, as his interest in the conversation quickened, his slow and hesitant speech became stronger, his laugh more vigorous, and his stooped frame appeared to straighten at the touch of the old energy that had driven his life.

Late in 1964 Clare became mortally ill. He entered the Toronto Western Hospital in November and died of metastatic carcinoma on 17 December 1964.

Chapter Thirteen

THE SUMMING-UP

What, in fact, was Clare Hincks's contribution to the mental health movement in Canada? For how much does he deserve credit? And what credit should be assigned to others?

His mental imbalance, with its fertile, active "ups" and depressing "downs" is central to his accomplishments. As a husband and father, Clare is somewhat of an enigma. He admitted that he always placed his work before his wife and children, and in the sense that he worked hard and was often absent from the home, this statement is true. Yet his first marriage lasted almost 40 years, ending only with the death of Mabel Millman Hincks. And he did provide some assistance in raising a family of three children, none of whom now appears visibly blighted by paternal rejection.

Clare never claimed that he alone founded the Canadian National Committee for Mental Hygiene, nor the mental hygiene movement in Canada. As Simmonds, the author of *From Asylum to Welfare*, has pointed out, many of the Ontario psychiatrists who participated so actively in the work of the CNCMH after its inception in 1918 had earlier been involved in a somewhat analogous organization, the Provincial Association for the Care of the Feeble-Minded. So reform was obviously in the air when Clare became active in the field.

The major sources of inspiration and support in the early years of Clare's mental hygiene work were C.K. Clarke and Clifford Beers. Not only did Beers' American organization provide the model for its Canadian counterpart, but Beers himself played an active role in the creation of the CNCMH in the early months of 1918. He spoke at fund-raising meetings, handed out copies of his book, and served as an informal consultant whom Clare often called upon.

Dr. Clarke's role in the mental hygiene movement is less easy to define. He was the outstanding psychiatrist in Canada at that time and, after 1916, was president of the Toronto branch of the Provincial Association for the Care of the Feeble-Minded. He undoubtedly knew of the National Committee in the USA, and may have recommended that Clare call on Beers in New York. Clare has acknowledged his debt to Clarke for his psychiatric education but implied that, rather than directing him to a specific career in mental hygiene, Clarke allowed him the opportunity to find his own niche. Whatever the facts, there is no reason to doubt that Clarke's backing was important, even decisive, in the rapid formation of the CNCMH in the spring of 1918.

The hard work, however, was done by Clare. We know of his fund-raising trips during February, March, and April of 1918. He was engaged full-time in mental hygiene work whereas Clarke's commitment to it was only one in a myriad of other activities and duties. He was Dean of the Faculty of Medicine, Professor of Psychiatry, and active on many committees and with other groups. In fact, his salary was provided by the CNCMH on a "piece-work" basis in the early years, a clear indicator of his part-time status. It was Hincks, not Clarke, who presented the first address to the Canadian Medical Association to introduce the CNCMH. And as early as June, 1918, just two months after the CNCMH was formed, Evelyn Molson Russel wrote in the *Canadian Medical Association Journal*, " ... it is to Doctor Clarence M. Hincks, of Toronto University, that we owe the co-ordination of effort which has resulted in our new Canadian National Committee for Mental Hygiene ...."

Clarke provided the influence of his name, the benefit of his broad knowledge in psychiatry, and his encouragement; Hincks, in turn, imported the basic idea from the USA, kindled interest, and forced action with his tireless enthusiasm. He was an energetic full-time worker for the movement and contributed his unique ability to mobilize sympathy and to convert it into the hard cash that paid the bills.

After 1924, Clare received directorial control of the CNCMH. From that time until the late 1940s, the Committee was molded as he thought appropriate, and great things were accomplished. That the organization and some of its goals changed in the 10 years before his death, reflected the strength and adaptability he had built into its foundation.

We could estimate the millions of dollars Clare raised to promote better mental health; we can observe a vigorous organization which is his legacy; but the most remarkable of his achievements are less tangible. The general public is now far more tolerant and sympathetic towards the mentally ill than it was in 1918, and Canadians with mental disorders today receive better treatment than their forebears of fifty years ago; Clarence Meredith Hincks, more than any other person, was responsible for these changes.

His recurrent mental illness decisively shaped his life's work. The impact of men's illnesses on their lives has often been the object of study and conjecture. In Clare's case there is no doubt that he had some form of mental disease; later in his life he confessed to it in a CBC radio broadcast, in a deliberate, calculated move. He hoped his listeners, realizing that he was successful despite his disorder, would accept others with mental illness as assets to the community. He wanted to convince the world that mental illness had not hampered his career. So persuasive was he that his listeners might have wondered if his affliction was not an advantage.

An example may show that public acceptance of mental illness has grown during this century. A recently retired Professor of Medicine at McMaster University has published an autobiography entitled *Not Always on the Level*. The author, Dr. Moran Campbell, who has had a distinguished career both in the United Kingdom and in Canada, has written his book partly to show that a severely manic-depressive individual can accomplish a great deal. Dr. Campbell is his own subject. He and Clare Hincks would have had much in common.

Clare first became aware of his mental problem at the age of sixteen or seventeen when he entered the University of Toronto. In his autobiographical notes, dictated in 1962, he stated that his mother, having helped him with school work all through public and high school, decided that he should work without her help when he reached university. Perhaps the pressure that resulted from this decision contributed to his first episode of illness.

He described his illness as recurrent bouts of inactivity coupled with a feeling of depression. The episodes, which occurred about once a year, lasted a few weeks and then vanished. There were no known suicide attempts during the "low" periods which, as Clare learned from the very first attack, were self-limited. On that occasion he went to bed and waited. In ten days or two weeks he felt better and returned to his studies. No physician examined him nor did he take any form of treatment. In later years many of his close friends, psychiatrists, attempted to help him. Yet his attacks did not change in character, and time remained their only certain cure.

How did he behave when he was not depressed? He perceived himself as "ill" when depressed and "normal" at all other times. Yet his capacity for prodigious work, between bouts of depression, was legendary among mental health workers in Canada. He travelled a great deal, mostly before the age of air travel. Every visit to city or town was a renewed challenge. He responded enthusiastically to challenge, not only accomplishing vast quantities of work himself, but also inspiring the local workers by the sheer force of his enthusiasm. An example of what he could accomplish in a short time, and perhaps the most relevant example possible, is his organizing the Canadian National Committee for Mental Hygiene in 1918. Before February, 1918, no similar organization had existed in Canada. The idea came to him from New York, but the backing of the medical profession was assured by the active co-operation of C.K. Clarke. Yet there is no doubt that it was Clarence Hincks's enthusiasm and hard work that brought the Canadian National Committee for Mental Hygiene into existence on 26 April 1918.

Can hard work, coupled with enthusiasm, be stigmatized as abnormal? Periodic changes in levels of activity, both physical and mental, are a universal experience. At one end of the emotional spectrum lies the black depression which may culminate in suicide. At the other, a restless mania which, by the rapidity and insistence of its ideas, blocks an ordered and coherent approach to the tasks of daily living. Between these easily recognizable extremes, the line which separates "normal" mood swings from the "abnormal" cannot be clearly defined.

Clare was incapacitated when depressed but he was not disabled while, in his active phase, he functioned at an exceptionally high emotional and intellectual level. He would wish to be remembered as a man who, as he himself publicly disclosed, suffered from a chronic, recurrent mental illness, but who, in spite of it, accomplished more than most. For the mentally ill and emotionally distressed, we can be thankful that he was more often active than depressed, zealous than despairing, and abundantly effective in translating his dreams into reality.

ENDNOTES

1. Later, in 1919, when Hincks, Beers and others were trying to form an International Committee for Mental Hygiene, Osler was approached as a prospective leader. However, his death in December of that year prevented such a possibility.

2. John Bunyan. *Jerusalem Sinner Saved, or Good News for the Vilest of Men*. 1688

3. *Canadian Journal of Mental Hygiene* 1:30, 1919.

4. *MENN* pp 635-636.

5. "Survey of the Province of Manitoba," *Canadian Journal of Mental Hygiene* 1:77, 1919.

6. Certainly Clare had Osler's sense if not the exact words; what Osler said in his address on "Science and Immortality" (1904) was: "Some of you will wander through all phases [of belief], to come at last, I trust, to the opinion of Cicero, who had rather be mistaken with Plato than be in the right with those who deny altogether the life after death; and this is my own *confessio fidei*."

BIBLIOGRAPHY

The following books and articles may be helpful to any reader who wishes more information about Dr. Hincks, the history of psychiatry in Canada, or the mental hygiene movement. The chief archival source of information on Hincks and on the CNCMH is the Queen Street Mental Health Centre Archives (Griffin-Greenland Collection), 1001 Queen St. West, Toronto, Ontario.

Beers, Clifford. *A Mind That Found Itself: An Autobiography.* First Published 1908. Garden City, NY: Doubleday, Doran and Co. Inc., 1935

Campbell, Moran. *Not Always on the Level.* Cambridge: Cambridge University Press, 1988.

Dain, Norman. *Clifford W. Beers: Advocate for the Insane*. Pittsburgh: University of Pittsburgh Press, 1980.

Greenland, Cyril. "Services for the mentally retarded in Ontario, 1870-1930," *Ontario History*. 54: 267-74, 1962.

-----. "The treatment of the mentally retarded in Ontario—an historical note," *Canadian Psychiatric Association Journal*. 8: 328-36, 1963.

-----. *Charles Kirk Clarke, A Pioneer of Canadian Psychiatry*. Toronto: Clarke Institute of Psychiatry, 1966.

Roland, Charles G. "Clarence Hincks in Manitoba, 1918," *Manitoba Medical Review*. 46: 107-113, 1966

Russel, C.M. "The origin, organization and scope of the Canadian National Committee for Mental Hygiene," *Canadian Medical Association Journal*. 8: 538-46, 1918.

Shortt, S.E.D. *Victorian Lunacy: Richard M. Bucke and the Practice of Late Nineteenth-Century Psychiatry*. Cambridge: Cambridge University Press, 1986.

Simmonds, Harvey G. *From Asylum to Welfare*. Downsview: National Institute on Mental Retardation, 1982.

LIST OF ILLUSTRATIONS

All illustrations are from the Hincks family collection except where otherwise noted.

Charcoal drawing of Clarence Hincks, M. D. by Harold Shaw, 1954 10

Cartoon which appeared in *Torontenensis*, p. 181, 1907
(courtesy of Dr. C.G. Roland) 20

Clarence Hincks, with his parents at Windermere,
Lake Rosseau, circa 1913 33

Mabel Millman, shortly before her marriage to Clarence Hincks, 1912 .. 34

Clarence Meredith Hincks, on Lake Muskoka, circa 1923 35

Back row: Barbara Hincks, Clarence Meredith Hincks; front row:
Mabel Hincks, William Hincks, and Margaret Hincks, June 1942 36

Mabel Hincks, probably late 1940s 73

Clarence Hincks, 1957 74

Clarence Hincks, Muskoka, summer 1964 75

C.M. Hincks Institute (courtesy of Audrey M. Wilson) 76

INDEX

Alexander, Emma, 106
Allen Memorial Institute, Montreal, 111
Althouse, John, 106
American Board of Psychiatry and Neurology, 100
American Medico-Psychological Association, 63
Anderson, George, 13, 81
Angus, R.B., 43
Armstrong, J.W., 54
Atkinson Charitable Foundation, 112
Atkinson, Joseph E., 29, 62

Banham, K., 68
Banting, Frederick, 11, 79
Bates, Gordon, 14
Beatty, Sir Edward W., 43-44, 108, 110
Bengough, J.W., 12
Bertram, James, 70
Binet-Simon intelligence tests, 30, 77, 110
Birkenhead, Lord, 85
Blake, Daniel, 105
Blatz, William, 68, 70, 81, 82 106, 107, 111
Bone, John, 30
Bott, Ned, 30, 68, 70, 81, 105
Bridges, J.W., 68
British National Council for Mental Hygiene, 88
Brown, J.N.E., 32
Bruce, Herbert, 21
Bucke, Richard Maurice, 11
Bullis, Edmund, 71, 98, 101-102
Burn, Sir George, 43
Burgess, T.J.W., 62-63

Campbell, Moran, 122
Canadian Mental Health Association, 43, 53, 109-10, 112-13, 117
Canadian National Committee for Mental Hygiene, 39, 43, 45-46, 52-55, 57, 62, 65, 67, 77, 80, 88-89, 95, 101, 104, 109, 120-21, 123
Canadian Psychiatric Association, 109
Carnegie Trust, 88
Carruthers, Lillian, 61
CBC, 109, 114, 122
Chambers, J.B., 49
Chandler, A.B., 69
Chant, Sperrin, 68
Chisholm, Brock, 104-05
Church, "Tommy", 67
Clarke, C.K., 31, 39, 44, 50, 59, 63, 65-66, 77, 92, 109, 115, 118, 123
Clarke, E. De V., 37, 118
Commonwealth Fund, 98
Cosgrave, Gerald, 80
Coué, Emile, 84-85
Cousins Fund, 106
Craig, Sir Morris, 85

Dafoe, Alan Roy, 14
Department of Public Health and Preventive Medicine, McGill University, 77
Devonshire, 9th Duke of, 42, 43
Dunlap, D.A., 43

Eaton, Jack, 111
Eaton, Lady Flora, 108
Ebaugh, Franklin, 99
Embree, Edward, 66-67, 87, 101
Eugenical Sterilization Act, 78

Falconer, Sir Robert, 66
Ferguson, Howard, 61
Fidlar, Eddie, 14
Fleming, Grant, 77, 110
Framingham Experiment, 92
Franks, Ruth, 105
Freud, Sigmund 68, 92, 94

Geel, Belgium, 94
Gesell, Arnold, 69
Goldsmith, Perry, 21, 22
Good, T.S., 92-93
Gooderham, G.H., 29
Graham, Duncan, 11
Griffin, Jack, 79, 82, 104-05, 110, 112, 114, 117

Halpenny, J., 46, 64
Halsam, John, 50
Hamilton, Samuel, 100
Hamlin, Fred, 23
Henderson, Ernest, 14
Hilliker, Kathleen, 113
Hincks, Barbara Mary, 35, 73, 116-17
Hincks, Mabel (Millman), 27, 35, 72-74, 79, 115-17, 120
Hincks, Margaret Maude, 35, 73, 108, 116-17
Hincks, Mattie (Greene), 11-13, 83
Hincks, Norman William, 72, 73, 116-17
Hincks, William Henry, 11, 83
Holden, John B., 43
Huntsman, Archie, 14, 16
Huxley, Thomas, 15

International Congress on Mental Hygiene, 114
IQ tests *see* Binet-Simon intellignece tests
Ittleson, Mrs. Henry, 98

Jacques, Hazel, 57-58
Jaffray, Stuart, 106-07
James, Canon, 79
James, William, 68
Jamieson, Sir Wilson, 106-07
Janet, Pierre, 91-92
Johnson, Melvin M., 101
Jones, Ernest, 32
Judge Baker Foundation, 81

Ketchum, David, 68, 71
Keyes, Marjorie, 37, 44, 46, 49, 77-78, 97, 98, 105, 113, 116, 118
Komora, Paul, 39
Kraepelin, Emil, 93-94
Kubie, Lawrence, 105

Lapp, R.E., 28
Laura Spellman Rockefeller Memorial Fund, 68, 70
Lawson, Frank, 80
LeBourdais, D.M., 110
Letson, H.F.G., 104
Line, William, 68, 77, 81-82, 104, 114
Lusk, C.S., 113

MacLeod, Stanley, 106
MacMurchy, Helen, 31-32
MacNeill, J.W., 57-58
MacPhee, E.D., 68
Manitoba
Brandon Hospital for the Insane, 49, 52
Psychopathic Hospital, 53-54
Publick Welfare Commission, 45-46, 51, 53-54
Selkirk Hospital for the Insane, 51
Maritime Home for Girls, 56-57
Martin, Charles F., 43-44, 87
Massey, Vincent, 43, 67
Mathers, A.T., 46, 54
Maudsley Address, 65
Mayo, Elton, 85, 91-92
McConnel, John, 108
McGill University, 41-42, 67, 68, 80, 86
McIllwraith, Kenneth, 22
McMurchie, Helen, 30-31
McPhedran, Alexander, 22
McPhedran, Fletcher, 14
Menninger, Karl, 38
Mental Diseases Act, 1919, 53-54
Mental Health Award, 118
Mental Health Week, 109
Mental Hygiene Institute, 68, 80, 118
Meredith, Sir Vincent, 43
Metcalfe, W.C., 59
Meyer, Adolph, 85
Millman, Norman, 13
Millman, Thomas, 115
Mitchell, Bert, 68, 80
Molson, F.W., 43
Molson Russel, Evelyn, 121
Mott, Hawley, 81
Mulholland, Ross, 14
Mundie, Gordon, 41
Murray, W.C., 57

National Film Board, 109
999 Queen Street, 32, 37
Nixon, H.C., 60, 62
No. 4 Canadian General Hospital, 37, 118
Noble, Ralph, 99

Ontario College of Education, 80
Ontario Educational Association, 60
Osler, Sir William, 16, 90
Osler, Sir Edmund, 67, 69
Osler, Featherstone, 69

Parks, J.D., 112-13
Parmenter, Morgan, 80
"Penny Roundup", 113
Peterson, William, 42
Potts, W.A., 85
Pratt, E.J., 30, 43
Price, William, 43
Provincial Association for the Care of the Feeble-Minded, 120-21
Pryce, James, 113
Psychiatric Clinic, Toronto, 41
Psychoanalysis, 92

Queen's Canadian Fund, 108

Reeve, Richard "Dicky", 21
Robertson, John Ross, 67
Rockefeller Foundation, 66-67, 83, 86, 88, 103
Rockwood Hospital, Kingston, 32, 59, 115
Royal Canadian Army Medical Corps, 21, 81, 104
Royal College of Physicians and Surgeons of Canada, 23, 100
Royal Victoria Hospital, 68
Ruml, Beardsley, 68
Russel, Colin K., 41, 45-46

Salmon, Thomas, 96
Scottish Rite Masons, 101
Seeley, Jack, 110
"Shacktown", 28
Shaughnessy, Thomas George, 1st Baron 43
Silverman, Baruch, 68, 80
Simmonds, H.G., 120
Slight, David, 68
Smith, Barry, 98, 100
Smith, Elliot, 65, 86, 92
Smith, W.G., 30, 64
Spaulding, Harry, 110
Starr, Judge, 31
Strothard, Josephine, 56-57

Thornton, R.S., 53
Toronto Star, 30, 40, 60, 62
Toronto General Hospital, 21-23, 31, 37, 64
Toronto Globe, 61
Toronto Hospital for the Insane, 32
Toronto Juvenile Court, 31, 80
Toronto Psychiatric Hospital, 67, 111
Toronto Religious Education Council, 117
Toronto Evening Telegram, 67

United States National Committee for Mental Hygiene, 96, 98
University of Toronto, 14, 64, 66-67-68, 70, 77, 80, 119

Warren, Mrs. H.D., 43
White Cross Open Door Service, 113
Williams, Frankwood, 39, 69, 96-98
Winnipeg General Hospital, 52
Withrow, O.C.J., 32, 37, 118
World Federation for Mental Health, 114
Wright, Ramsay, 15